GRANDPARENTS AS PARENTS

GRANDPARENTS AS PARENTS

A Survival Guide for Raising a Second Family

Sylvie de Toledo
Deborah Edler Brown

Foreword by Ethel Dunn

THE GUILFORD PRESS
New York / London

© 1995 Sylvie de Toledo and Deborah Edler Brown
Written by Deborah Edler Brown

Published by The Guilford Press
A Division of Guilford Publications, Inc.
72 Spring Street, New York, NY 10012

The following copyright holders have generously given permission
to reprint from previously published works:
   Charlotte Observer for quotations from "When Grandparents Start
Over" by Miriam Durkin. Copyright 1991 by *Charlotte Observer*.
Used by permission.
   Ethel Dunn for a quotation from "Those Wonderful Abuelas" in
Intergenerational Hookup. Copyright 1993 by Ethel Dunn. Used
by permission.
   Grandparents United for Children's Rights, Inc., for suggestions
from *A Walk Through Policyland*. Copyright 1991 by Grandparents
United for Children's Rights, Inc. Used by permission.
   Senior Highlights for quotations from "Grandmothers Fill In for
Drug-Abusing Parents" by Miriam Dobbin. Copyright 1990 by *Senior
Highlights*. Used by permission.
   U.S. News & World Report for a quotation from "Silent Saviors"
by Linda L. Creighton. Copyright 1991 by *U.S. News & World
Report*. Used by permission.

Printed in the United States of America

This book is printed on acid-free paper.

Last digit is print number: 9   8   7   6   5   4   3   2   1

Library of Congress Cataloging-in-Publication Data

de Toledo, Sylvie.
      Grandparents as parents : a survival guide for raising a second
   family / Sylvie de Toledo and Deborah Edler Brown.
         p.   cm.
      Includes bibliographical references and index.
      ISBN 1-57230-011-6. — ISBN 1-57230-020-5 (pbk.)
      1. Grandparent and child.   2. Child rearing.   3.
   Intergenerational relations.   I. Brown, Deborah Edler.   II.
   Title.
   HQ759.9.D423   1995
   649'.1—dc20   95-19656
                                                         CIP

To the memory of Nikki de Toledo;
her son, Kevin;
and Andre and Ginette, the grandparents who raised him

To grandparents everywhere
who are struggling to protect their grandchildren

We bereaved are not alone. We belong to the largest company in all the world—the company of those who have known suffering. When it seems that our sorrow is too great to be borne, let us think of the great family of the heavy-hearted into which our grief has given us entrance, and, inevitably, we will feel about us their arms, their sympathy, their understanding.

—Helen Keller

Foreword

The following excerpt is from a letter that I recently received from a grandmother named Charlotte, who catapulted out of the ranks of grandparenthood into that of surrogate parent early one September morning:

> *It's 12:00 midnight. A few minutes ago as I walked down the hall toward the kitchen to get myself a glass of water I glanced at my 4½-year-old grandson sleeping peacefully in his bedroom and thought how different our lives were now from only a short time ago.*
>
> *Calvin's mother brought him to me at 3:00 A.M. the morning of 9/7/92. He arrived with no food; neither did she bring extra clothes. There he stood, a bewildered, scared little boy dressed in a pair of blue jeans with about ten holes in them, no underwear, a shirt that was much too big for his little body, and a pair of dirty white bedroom slippers. She told me that he was my grandchild. We didn't know each other. He was 17 months old when she left without any word. She asked if I would keep him until the following weekend when she would come back for him.*
>
> *That weekend and many more have come and gone without any word from her. Calvin and I are doing fine because we have each other. We get by on my small Social Security check. We don't know where his mother is. I've gotten an order for temporary custody that allows me to take him to the doctor if he gets sick, and I will put him in school next month. But where is his mother? Will she ever return, and if she does, what will happen to Calvin then?*
>
> *Please help me. I need some answers and direction.*

Grandparents throughout the ages have served as support for their children and grandchildren, and generational interdependence has long been a significant part of American society. The major difference between past generations and the current one, however, is that in the past—except in the event of the death of a parent—grandparents tended to be ancillary in furnishing support to their children's families. Although they certainly provided goods and services to enhance the young family, they, for the most part, assumed a background role in the actual parenting of the children.

Historical tradition has changed, however, and many of today's grandparents now find themselves long- or short-term parents again. Often, they must adjust to being part of a nontraditional family in which parental roles may be reversed: parents may become virtual siblings, aunts, or other kin; parents may not be in the picture at all; or grandparents may have to become parents. Confusion reigns, not only on the part of the children but also in the minds of their caregivers/surrogate parents.

It is to this group of dedicated and caring people that the immensely useful and impressive book you are about to read is directed: the millions of "Charlotte(s)" who daily give of themselves so that their grandchildren may live with love and compassion and without fear of abandonment.

Only a few years ago, little was said about grandparents raising their grandchildren. Today, largely because of social advocacy, we see more media coverage of these circumstances, and we know now that our numbers are large and growing, and that this growth is expected to continue.

What is often not reflected in the media, however, is how grandparent caregivers and their young charges are getting along. What are they feeling, and how are they coping? What are their major concerns and desires? What forms of help do they need when they reach out for support, and what agencies or persons are best equipped to bolster them in times of need? Finally, two people have come along to put some answers to these questions.

When grandparent advocate Sylvie de Toledo first discussed the idea of a book for grandparents who are raising their grandchildren, I was very exctied. I knew that she was just the person who could speak to this audience with empathy and kindness, but also with amazing firmness. I understood that if anyone could offer grandparents a sense of direction it would be Sylvie. From time to time over the three years that it took to complete the book, either she or writer Deborah Edler Brown would call and read half-finished sections to me for input. I have now read the completed book, and can truthfully say that my initial hopes have been surpassed.

What you are about to begin is a reference book that reads like a novel. It is poetic, gentle, and thoughtful, and yet it is brimming with vital information—no page can be skipped.

Furthermore, *Grandparents as Parents: A Survival Guide for Raising a Second Family* could only have been conceived of by someone who has been through the trauma of a family broken by tragedy, by one who has chosen to be there for others who need help and direction. Its availability offers us hope, and validates our personal fears, angers, frustrations, and pain. It points us toward sanity and reason in the face of dilemma and need. We are taken, step by painful step, through the process of learning again how to function as a parent, especially in these complicated times. We are retaught old skills and trained in the process of learning new ones. No topic is too insignificant or cumbersome to be examined, either succinctly or in a thorough manner. Our own personal needs and those of the children that we love and cherish are examined openly and in a straightforward manner.

This remarkable book can be used as a resource not only by those courageous many who have assumed the responsibilities of parenting, loving, and nurturing a generation of potentially lost children, but also by those who serve them—our social service personnel, family therapists, legal professionals, and any others who work cross-generationally with families to help them stay whole.

Ethel Dunn
Executive Director,
Grandparents United for Children's Rights

Acknowledgments

No book of this scope can come to light without the support of a number of people—friends and family, sources, and many outside experts who patiently offered insight and clarification. From the moment this project was conceived to the time the final manuscript was set, we have been graced with heartfelt enthusiasm and help from some very wonderful individuals.

Our first thanks must go to our families for their boundless support and encouragement, particularly our parents, Andre and Ginette de Toledo, Jack Brown and Ana Edler Brown, Sylvie's brother and sister-in-law, Philip and Alyce, Deborah's brother Arthur, and Sylvie's nephew Kevin, who has been very open in sharing his story. Words do not adequately express how deeply they have all affected the success of this project. From the beginning of *Grandparents as Parents*, the program and the book, Sylvie's family members have been case studies, cheerleaders, reseach assistants, volunteers, benefactors, and all-around silent partners. From the beginning of the book project, Deborah's family has been a sounding board, an editorial board, and an ongoing pep rally. Indeed, special credit must go to Deborah's brother Arthur, who carefully read and helped trim an overgrown manuscript with exquisite insight and precision. Our families have offered praise, advice, warm meals, strong shoulders, and even grants when times were lean. We could not have done this book without them.

We owe much to our wonderful editor Kitty Moore. From start to finish, she has been a guide through unfamiliar terrain, a deft ambassador between authors and publisher, and an expert coach whose enthusiasm and clear understanding focused our vision. A similar vote of thanks goes to Wendy Ross, whose preliminary editing helped strengthen and shape the architecture of a complex subject.

JoBeth McDaniel was our matchmaker for this project. An accomplished journalist herself, JoBeth wrote the original proposal for this book but was prevented from actually writing it due to prior commitments. Instead, she eagerly introduced us to each other, and a happy meeting it was. If books have godmothers, JoBeth would be ours.

We have been graced with guardian angels as well. We are indebted to attorneys Larry Hanna, Pamela Mohr, Michael Salazar, Yolanda Vera, Peter Wright, and Ted Youmans, who have shared their time, knowledge, and resources to help us anchor this book in practical, accurate information about family law, government aid, and special education. All have made time in their overcommitted schedules to read drafts of chapters and clarify subtle shifts of meaning. They have also been on call to answer the numerous tiny, detailed questions that came up in the last pressured moments of rewriting. We are equally grateful to Samuel Hananel, Phil Hopkins, Stephen Poe, and Richard Sherer for jumping in as ad hoc editors, proofreaders, and consultants at several critical junctures, offering their expertise and enthusiasm; to Sheila Milnes for her insight on issues of childrearing; and to Pamela Darr Wright for her help in unraveling the IEP process.

We also wish to thank Jacqueline Battle, Alice Bussiere, Leza Davis, Charles Ollinger, Anne Rutherford, Lori Waldinger, Dana Wilson, the ADD+ Forum at CompuServe, and the Department of Health and Human Services and the helpful people who work there. They have all extended themselves to ensure that valuable information reaches the hands of families in need.

Thanks to Karen and Heidi Toffler, as well as Ken Stuckey from the Perkins School for the Blind, for doggedly tracking down the source of the marvelous quote from Helen Keller that starts the book; to Stuart Chapin, for offering up Carl Sandburg as a way to end it; and to Alvin Toffler for his lessons on how to put it all together.

Many others have helped out in quiet but important ways. Deborah would like to thank the close friends and extended family who have offered support, counsel, hugs, and incredible patience with the mental and physical absences of a writer in labor. In addition to those already mentioned, special thanks go to Joe Anthony, Diane Davidson, Josh Gambin, Greg Hughart, Claudia Kazachinsky, Keli Morgan, Kaliko Orian, Donna Pall, Marianne Simon, Andrew Stein, Andrea Trisciuzzi, and Kaki Woods, as well as to Richard Wells, who helped nurture a love of words, to the Browns and the Edlers for funding the first computer, and to Sarah Crane, who so graciously tolerated the wayward schedule of her Aunt Deb.

Of course, none of this would have come together without the wonderful people at The Guilford Press. We thank them for their dedicated work, their enthusiasm, and their patience with frantic phone calls from new authors. We particularly appreciate the careful work of the book's production editor at Guilford, Anna Brackett, and the copyediting of Toby Troffkin. We are grateful to our art director, Ty Cumbie, for giving our book such a beautiful face, and to Lyn Grossman, Rowena Howells, Lori Rothstein, Keisha Simmons, and Kitty Stewart for their parts in turning a manuscript into a book. We also want to thank assistant marketing director Anne Newman for her belief that this is an important book and publicist Phyllis Heller for making sure that people see it.

It's hard to find the right words to describe Ethel Dunn. Friend, colleage, advocate, grandmother, Ethel's exuberance was like food and fresh air when we were weary. She gave us perspective, information, and let us read fledgling chapters to her long-distance. She also lent us her own talents as a writer by writing the foreword to this book. Her excitement has been invaluable.

We are particularly grateful to the past and present board members of Grandparents As Parents (GAP): Carole Bloom, Barbara Castro, Rosalie Cauley, Florence Gilmore, Judith Hirsch, Betty Linstead, Joan McMillin, and Barbara Wasson. There is no way to measure what they have given of themselves in time, money, energy, and heart, to promote the cause of grandparents. They have been our staunchest cheering section, and we couldn't have gotten this far without them.

We deeply appreciate the efforts of all the journalists and talk show hosts who are shedding light on grandparent issues and of all the advocates who are working to improve the plight of grandparents and of children in general.

Finally, no thanks would be complete without remembering the countless grandparents who have so generously shared their stories with us. It was their faces, and the faces of their grandchildren, that kept us going in the bleak hours when the road seemed too long and writing one more word seemed like an inhuman task. They were our humanity, and our light.

Contents

Introduction

In 1983 my sister committed suicide. She locked the doors of her house and overdosed on pills that had been prescribed for depression. She didn't leave a note. She did leave an eight-year-old son. She was 27 years old.

I was away in graduate school, finishing a master's degree in social work. My sister and I had a standing phone date. Every Saturday morning at six o'clock I would call her. My nephew would be asleep, and we could talk without interruption. As a single mother, my sister didn't have much time without interruption. Since Kevin would wake up at some point during the call, I would talk to him, too. Nikki and I were close in age—one year and one week apart—and we were best friends.

That Saturday I called and called, but there was no answer. I finally called my parents to see if they knew where Nikki was. Kevin had spent the previous night at my brother's house and was scheduled to stay with my parents that night to give his mother a free weekend. But she hadn't said anything about going out. We decided they should use the spare key and go in. It didn't work. One lock wouldn't open. It was the one Nikki locked from inside. "She's in there, Mom," I said. "I know she's in there." My parents had the police knock down the door. Nikki was there, but it was too late. I caught the next plane to Los Angeles (by this time, it was early the next morning).

Overnight, we went from a family of five adults to one of four, a hand with a missing finger. We were devastated, and we were in shock. Grief had joined our family.

And then there was Kevin.

Kevin had always been the family child. Nikki dropped out of school at 18 to have him. His father was never part of the picture.

1

And although Nikki and Kevin had their own apartment, my parents, my brother, and I were always helping out in different ways. Kevin was lovable and he was difficult. Now, at the age of eight, he was parentless.

There was no question of what to do. My parents took Kevin in, and in that moment they became part of a family much larger than ours, although we didn't know it then. They joined the growing ranks of grandparents who are raising their grandchildren.

The media calls them "silent saviors,"[1] "recycled parents,"[2] and, when they are also caring for aging parents, "the sandwich generation."[3] At a time in their lives when they expected to be traveling, enjoying hobbies, and doing everything they had put on hold while raising their first set of children, they find themselves back in a routine of bottles, diapers, and PTA meetings, sometimes 30 years after they last had kids in the house. Instead of doting grandparents who can spoil and coddle and send the kids back to Mom and Dad, they are surrogate parents with all the responsibilities of raising another set of children.

Some are as young as 35, others are in their 70s. Some are even great-grandparents and step-grandparents. They cross economic lines, social lines, and religious lines. They become caregivers because of abandonment, neglect, and abuse, as well as death by illness, accident, suicide, and murder. In some instances their adult children are in jail or mentally ill. By far, the most common reason grandparents raise grandchildren is parental drug and alcohol abuse.

The kids these grandparents get are troubled, burdened with everything from emotional, behavioral, psychological, medical, and academic problems to physical disabilities from a parent's prenatal drug and alcohol abuse.

More than three million children live in the homes of their grandparents. Even so, too many grandparents think they are in this alone. Not a day goes by that I don't get phone calls and letters from grandparents around the country who are looking for a group, a piece of information, or someone to listen to them who will understand their concerns. The letters come typed, written, and scribbled in crayon, on everything from napkins to torn scraps of paper. Some write "Dear Ms. de Toledo" or "Dear GAP [Grandparents As Parents]" and tell their stories; others just write "Help!" One grandparent in Georgia seemed to say it for all of them when he wrote, "I took my grandson when his mother died six years ago.

Ten months ago, his dad died. We need people. My friends call once in a while but don't come around. We are like in a world alone. We need people."

This book had to be done because there was absolutely nothing out there to answer those letters. I talked to thousands of grandparents across the country and realized there was nothing to help these families. People asked me about resources, and because I had nowhere to refer them, I would offer to help start a group in their community.

Before I started my first Grandparents As Parents support group in 1987, I searched a number of libraries for information on grandparents raising grandchildren. I was looking for a foundation. If there was material out there, I didn't want to reinvent the wheel. Unfortunately, I didn't find anything in the professional literature, let alone the consumer press.

Since then, GAP has grown into an organization of nine support groups across southern California and has helped start hundreds of others throughout the country. Local grandparent groups across the United States have joined forces to create a strong national voice on grandparent issues. Various organizations have created pamphlets, brochures, and newsletters. Researchers have just begun to study the grandparenting phenomenon, and a few authors have published books on the changing role of grandparents.[4] Still, there is nothing out there that addresses the broad spectrum of grandparent issues in one place.

So, this is *GAP: The Book.* It is part map, part dictionary, and something of a group hug—a handbook for all grandparents who are raising grandchildren, to help them through the stressful times. Inside you will find descriptions of many of the common problems grandparents face when they take in their grandchildren, as well as practical suggestions for how to cope. You will also find basic information on topics such as government aid, court proceedings, and special education. I hope this book will help get you through the alphabet soup of AFDC, IEP, WIC, and CPS. In these pages you will find guidelines for forming groups and becoming politically active, two sure ways of empowering yourself in a situation that can often make you feel powerless. Here, as in a GAP meeting, I offer support, resource information, and a professional perspective. But it is the other grandparents who will let you know you are not alone, that you can get through this, that whatever you are going through is normal. In the following pages, you will hear their voices and their stories.*

Second-time parenting can be pretty grim sometimes. You face troubled children, uncooperative parents, and a bureaucracy that may not understand your new role or support your new needs. This book does not shy away from those stark realities. It does not suggest that if you follow a prescribed set of steps, your problems will vanish. Life isn't that simple. It does, however, offer hope. By raising grand-children, you offer them a new future. By learning your options you give yourself choices. By recognizing problems you learn when to adapt and when to fight back. And by joining forces you create hope for the grandparents who follow you.

A NOTE TO PROFESSIONALS WHO WORK WITH GRANDPARENTS

I hope this book will also provide insight for people who work with grandparents: mental health professionals, teachers, doctors, attor-neys—anyone who comes in contact with grandparents raising grand-children and children being raised by their grandparents.

I receive frequent requests from educators and mental health pro-fessionals on how to develop groups for grandparents. My work is based on years of observations of and therapeutic work with grandparent families, as well as on personal experience with my own family. This treatment incorporates many aspects: crisis intervention, individual needs assessment, meeting survival needs of individual families, model-ing coping skills, teaching problem-solving techniques, and supportive therapy. Some of the work I do is nontraditional for mental health professionals, but I believe it is critical for grandparent families.

Chapter 14 specifically addresses support groups for grandpar-ents: how to find them, how to start them, and what programs and principles have been successful for GAP. The chapter is designed to assist both grandparents and mental health professionals in the rewarding process of developing groups; I hope it helps you.

---

*So as to avoid using sexist language—and so as not to encumber it with an excessive use of "he or she" and "him or her"—we have decided to alternate between masculine and feminine pronouns. We have attempted to do this consistently, and have tried to avoid ascribing the male and female pronouns in a stereotypical way.

HOW TO READ THIS BOOK

Grandparents as Parents is designed as both a book and a manual. You can read it front to back, following the grandparent stories that span the chapters, or you can turn to whatever chapter addresses your immediate questions, without worrying about order.

The book is divided into three sections. Section I, "When the Second Shift Arrives," covers the personal and social aspects of raising grandchildren: the changes, the feelings, and the problems of adult children, grandchildren, and family in general. It starts with an overview of the recent rise in grandparents as parents and looks at some of the myths about the phenomenon. Section II, "Through the Red Tape," addresses the bureaucratic part of raising grandchildren, the legal issues, and the availability of government assistance and special education. And Section III, "Strength in Numbers," focuses on the larger community of grandparents as parents and provides information on finding and starting support groups as well as on the political aspects of the grandparent movement.

Grandparents as Parents represents the work of two authors—myself and journalist Deborah Edler Brown—yet it is written from one point of view. The reason is simple: We wanted this to be a comfortable, personal book, and ten years of working with grandparents has given me an intimate understanding of the subject. As you read through the following chapters, the voice and perspective you encounter will be mine. I hope they help you.

When my sister ended her life, a whole world ended for me. And another one opened. Somehow, when I see the growth of GAP, I feel that something positive is coming from the death of my sister. There is a special place in my heart for grandparents who are parenting again. You all deserve a gold medal for what you're doing. You have sacrificed to be here, and my heart goes out to you.

SYLVIE DE TOLEDO

Grandparents as Parents accurately conveys the themes that are the most central to grandparents who are raising grandchildren, but the names and identifying characteristics of most of the grandparents and grandchildren mentioned in the book have been changed in order to protect their privacy.

When the Second Shift Arrives

CHAPTER 1

Unplanned Parenthood: Why Me?

Becoming a parent again is not a first choice. It's
a last alternative.
—*Barbara Kirkland, founder
of Grandparents Raising Grandchildren*[1]

S ometimes the call comes at night, sometimes
on a bright morning. It may be your child,
the police, or child protective services.
"Mama, I've messed up. . . ." "We're sorry. There has been an
accident. . . ." "Mrs. Smith, we have your grandchild. Can you take
him?" Sometimes you make the call yourself—reporting your own
child to the authorities in a desperate attempt to protect your grandchild from abuse or neglect. Often the change is gradual. At first
your grandchild is with you for a day, then four days, a month, and
then two months as the parents slowly lose control of their lives.
You start out baby-sitting. You think the arrangement is temporary.
You put off buying a crib or moving to a bigger apartment. Then you
get a collect call from jail—or no call at all.

But whether the arrival is slow or sudden, at some point it
dawns on you: You are no longer watching your grandchildren, you
are raising them. Take the *grand* out of *grandparent*; you are parenting again, and your life will never be the same.

Emily Petersen knew her pregnant daughter-in-law, Sheila, was
a drug addict. She knew the young woman was using drugs throughout her entire pregnancy, and she was prepared to see the effects

in her newborn granddaughter—the stiff body, the frantic eyes, the shakes. What Emily was not prepared for was becoming a mother again at 59. But when she and her husband, Carter, arrived at the hospital to see the baby, they found a social worker and two body-guards outside the hospital room. Sheila had been arrested on drug charges, and the baby was being removed. The social worker asked Emily if she would be willing to take the child. "I came in to visit a baby," Emily told her. "I didn't come to take a baby home." But her son was in tears, begging them not to send Amanda into foster care, and neither Emily nor Carter could stand the idea of not knowing where their granddaughter was. A week later they filed for custody.

Ivy Johnson had not seen her daughter Rachel in four years; she had never even met her youngest granddaughter. They lived in Arizona and had no money to travel. Then Rachel left her husband and came home with her kids. The minute she came to the door, Ivy knew something more was wrong. Within three days Rachel was diagnosed with liver cancer. Seven months later she died, leaving Ivy to raise five young grandchildren in a one-bedroom apartment.

There is nothing new about a grandparent raising a child in a crisis. For centuries grandparents have taken over when their grandchildren were orphaned by disease or war or when financial troubles split a family. They have also stepped in to support single mothers and widowed or divorced parents of both sexes. Moreover, there is a proud tradition of intergenerational families in working-class neighborhoods as well as in African-American and Hispanic communities of all income levels.[2]

What *is* new are the numbers: of grandparents, of grandchildren, of crises. According to the U.S. Census Bureau, approximately 3.2 million children[3] under 18 were living in grandparents' homes in 1990—a 40 percent increase[4] in 10 years. Nearly one million homes had no parents present at all.[5] And the real numbers are probably higher: Many grandparents don't acknowledge or recognize that they are taking full-time care of their grandchildren; perhaps they only watch them four days a week or are ashamed to admit that their own children can't parent. Many don't believe the situation is permanent. Some estimates put the number of grandparents raising grandchildren at over five percent of American families.[6] That would be approximately 1 in 20 households, or one family per average city block. "What's wrong with my generation that we can't or won't raise our kids?" asks one young mother in Texas. The answer paints a picture of growing tragedy in American families.

AMERICA'S CHILDREN IN CRISIS

Grandparents raise grandchildren for one reason: because the children need someone to raise them. It was true a hundred years ago, and it is true today. Certainly, there are grandparents who try to "steal" their grandchildren, but the vast majority had other plans for this stage of their lives; raising another child wasn't part of them. To quote a grandmother in Oregon: "The bottom line of this whole thing is I didn't need another child; the child needed a mother."

On the other hand, there are many reasons why these children need their grandparents. One writer pinned the cause on what he called the four Ds: drugs, divorce, desertion, and the death of a parent.[7] Indeed, illness, accident, suicide, and murder leave numerous children without parents to care for them, and drugs and alcohol shatter thousands of young families each year. But child abuse, incarceration, joblessness, teen pregnancy, and now AIDS also contribute to the growing number of children without stable homes. Most families suffer from a combination of problems, and the rate at which all these problems are growing is frightening. The statistics point to a nation of children in crisis:

- One in two marriages ends in divorce. Nearly one million children experience divorce each year.[8] Some parents go on to remarry with little interest in their own offspring.
- Teen pregnancy rates are high.[9] Half a million children are born to teenagers in the United States each year.[10]
- Reports of child abuse and neglect are up 300% nationally since 1976.[11]
- The prison population has exploded. Eighty percent of inmates—men and women—are parents of dependent children.[12]
- More wome are using drugs, especially crack cocaine.[13] Every year 375,000 babies are born with drugs in their system.[14]
- AIDS is taking its toll on American families. Nearly 125,000 children will have lost their mothers to the disease by the year 2000.[15]

Many of these children end up in foster care, separated from their siblings and cared for by strangers. But the foster care system itself is in crisis, with a rising demand for care and a shrinking number of qualified foster parents. In some cities, public health officials have talked about a return to orphanages.[16]

All this leaves grandparents, and other relatives, as one of the few buffers between these children and an increasingly precarious future. In fact, as of 1994, 54 percent of children placed out of home in Los Angeles County were placed with grandparents and other relative caregivers.[17]

Whether your grandchild lives with you because of drugs, death, abuse, or abandonment, there are certain factors that are *not* responsible for this second parenthood, despite what people think.

THE MYTHS

There are several reactions that appear, like clockwork, each time a discussion turns to grandparents as parents. They are assumptions that allow people to explain away the phenomenon, to pretend that it doesn't touch them, and to put the blame, somehow, on the victim:

"It's a black problem, right?"
"It's a poor problem—or an urban problem—isn't it?"
"Well, those grandparents probably deserve it if they messed up their first set of kids."

These biases exist as much in the judge deciding a custody case as in the person watching the news. They are responsible for much of the intolerance you may encounter as you try to find help for yourself and protection for your grandkids. These assumptions imply that the "grandparenting" phenomenon is something that happens to someone else, when the sad truth is that each and every grandparent is only one or two tragedies away from the decision to raise a grandchild.

If you and the children you care for are ever to receive the help you desperately need and deserve, we must look through these myths and face head-on the incredible depth and scope of grandparents as parents.

Myth 1: It's an Urban, Minority Problem

Say "grandparents as parents" to people, and, for many, certain pictures come to mind: Black faces. Brown faces. City-dwellers. Families in poverty. These pictures are not inaccurate, but they are incomplete. Raising grandchildren is not strictly an urban, poor, or African-American problem. If it were, it would be no less of a social crisis. But it is not. It is a national problem.

Parenting a grandchild is a necessity born of tragedy, and tragedy has no regard for race, class, ethnicity, location, or religion. Grandparents are raising grandchildren in places as different from one another as New York City, Honolulu, and Paducah, Kentucky. Articles on second-time parenting have appeared in publications as diverse as the *Boston Globe*, the *Katy Times* (in Katy, Texas), the *Cleveland Jewish News*, and a local newsletter in Pottowattamie County, Iowa. More than half of these children are white, and nearly half are African-American,[18] and while Hispanic and other races represent the smallest numbers, they still account for 415,000 children.[19] Grandparenting is color-blind. It is also class-blind. The same can be said of the drug epidemic that drives it.

Drugs and alcohol account for more than 80 percent of grandparent families. They show up combined with teen pregnancy, abuse, neglect, and abandonment. They show up in connection with incarceration and murder. Moreover, suburban, middle-class, and white families are not immune from addiction; they only hide it better. Middle-class addicts may have better access to private drug treatment programs and may be less likely to end up in jail. Private doctors are less likely to question pregnant women about drugs and alcohol than are inner-city doctors in public clinics and county hospitals; private hospitals are also less likely to test pregnant women or newborns for drug exposure.[20]

According to a 1989 study by the National Association for Perinatal Addiction Research and Education (NAPARE), white women are just as likely to use cocaine, heroin, or marijuana during a pregnancy as black women, but black women are ten times more likely to be reported to the authorities.[21] "Physicians were selecting out those women who they perceived as drug abusers to test those babies and then reporting them through the system," says NAPARE president Ira Chasnoff.[22] To quote one grandmother, "Drugs affect us all, whether you live in the streets or in a mansion."

So does tragedy. Both are indiscriminate. Who you are and where you live are not to blame for your situation, and neither are you.

Myth 2: It's Your Fault

Diane Warner is a grandparent activist and founder of Second Time Around Parents in Pennsylvania. She is raising the son of a drug-addicted daughter. It is not uncommon in her lobbying work for her to hear this question: "If you have raised a drug addict, how can we trust you not to raise this child as a drug addict?"[23] It is a question grandparents hear all the time. It is a question that hangs in the air, spoken or unspoken. It floats through the legal system, where judges and social workers question the wisdom of placing children with their grandparents, wondering to what extent the grandparents are responsible for the adult child's inability to parent.

Similar questions haunt many grandparents themselves: "What did we do wrong?" "Is this our fault?" "Are we grandparenting because we failed as parents?" One grandmother feels guilty because she worked nights as a nurse; she fears that may be why her daughter is on drugs. Another is afraid that she didn't love her son enough, that maybe she wasn't there when he needed her and that it drove him to drugs.

Let me set the record straight.* You did not raise your children to be drug addicts, welfare mothers, prostitutes, or even irresponsible parents. Did you make mistakes in childrearing? Probably. Most people do. Are there things you could have done differently? Certainly. We all have 20/20 hindsight. But you did not cause your child's addiction or the abuse or neglect of his or her own child. You did the best you could with what you knew at the time. Again and again, I see families where two or three children grow up to be upstanding citizens and competent parents and one loses control of her life. The New Jersey grandparents who raised a talented musician, a successful accountant, and a young woman who became addicted to drugs. The Montana grandparents who raised three boys: an architect, a county sheriff, and a drug addict. How are these grandparents to be blamed for their children's failings?

---

*Please note that although this book represents the work of two authors, it is written from the point of view of one—Sylvie de Toledo.

Even when child abuse or addiction seems to run in a family—and these problems can be cyclical—grown people have a choice about whether to continue the cycle or break it. There are many adults who were abused as children who do not grow up to be abusers and many children of addicts who take a different path.

Again, the statistics are telling. The recent surge in grandparents raising grandchildren—a 40 percent increase—occurred between 1980 and 1990. That almost precisely coincides with the growth of the crack epidemic. But few grandparents knew much about marijuana, let alone cocaine, when they were raising children. And if you had known, what could you have done? When they caught their teenagers with marijuana, many grandparents marched them off to police stations only to have them slapped on the wrist and sent home. Moreover, many people experimented with drugs and alcohol as teenagers and grew up to be productive adults and parents. Besides, the truth is that most of the grandparents I see are not raising the children of teenagers. In fact, according to one expert, the average age for a crack mother is 25 to 28, and many are in their 30s.[24] "It is the use of substance that creates substance abuse problems," says California psychologist Michael Jones. "We have a whole society that has problems with that, and that is certainly not the making of any particular grandparent."[25]

No one makes a person take drugs, abandon a baby, or abuse a child. Whatever choices you made as parents are past you. You did the best you could. Your children are now adults, and they are making their own choices.

THE REASONS FOR GRANDPARENTING

There are many complicated reasons why grandchildren need grandparents to care for them. But, in the end, the reasons you take them in are straightforward and simple: love, duty, and the bonds of family. Over and over I hear the same refrains: "We want to keep the kids together." "We're all he has." Often you are the only one standing between your grandchild and foster care. I have seen many grandparents disrupt their lives, their finances, and their health to keep their grandchildren together and away from care by strangers.

Anne Sutter's grandson Gregory was born in a crack house, and his mother was arrested on drug-related charges. At 60 years of age and on a limited income, Anne was not prepared to care for an infant, but there was that tiny baby, born stiff and distorted, with drugs in his system, and Anne couldn't say no. She recalls, "I looked at him and thought to myself, 'Nobody else will love my baby; they will look at him and think he's a thing.'"

"Some of our friends say we're crazy, that they would never do this," another grandmother told a reporter. "But if we hadn't done this, in 15 years there might have been a knock on our front door and a young man standing there saying, 'I'm your grandson. Where were you when I needed you, when I lay in bed at night crying for someone to help me?'"[26]

A grandfather calls it a labor of love: "I don't think I could live with it if they went to somebody else."

CHAPTER 2

Taking Immediate Action

I live with my grandma because my mom left me on a hotel bench to go get a cup of coffee. You're not supposed to leave babies by theirselves.
—*Erica, age seven*

Late one Saturday night the phone call came: Leah Croft's 18-month-old grandson had been left unattended in an apartment. The little boy had tried to feed himself dry oatmeal and had started choking. Someone had called the police, and child protective services had removed the baby from his mother. They wanted Leah to take him in. Leah was already raising her daughter Jill's six-year-old twins but, because of Jill's transient lifestyle, had only seen her grandson three times before that night. At 10:30 P.M., Josh arrived in the arms of a social worker. Dressed in a sleeper that had the legs cut off because it was too small for him, he had no socks, no shoes, no bottle, no car seat, and only the diaper he was wearing. The next day was a frenzy. In addition to buying baby supplies, Leah had to find a sitter so she could go to work Monday morning. She had to buy diapers with her credit card because she didn't have enough cash. No one from social services told her she was eligible for government aid for the baby, and when she called to ask about it, she got the runaround. "For five months I didn't get one dime," she fumes. "Not one dime!"

Whether a grandchild arrives in one night or over a period of months, few grandparents plan, anticipate, or prepare for a second parenthood. Your home and lifestyle are geared to adult living. You are not expecting these children or these changes. Instead of one small baby, you may, like Ivy Johnson, acquire several children at once, all at different ages with different needs. Instead of the assured rights of parents, you may find that as grandparents you have no legal right to care for the children you are battling on all fronts to protect. Moreover, you may find your resources tapped in the process. As a grandparent raising grandchildren, you are facing complex emotional, financial, and legal situations that you are rarely prepared for. You may have to resolve problems overnight that most parents address over a period of months, if not years. While each family has different needs, there are a few things that every grandparent should look into as soon as possible:

▪ *Consider other options.* Some grandparents don't have the health or resources to raise a second family, but they do it anyway. A few, however, have been able to place their grandchild with another family member, perhaps a son or daughter who already had children and was willing to raise this child as well. If you have family members who can help out, you might consider letting them step in or at least sharing the responsibility with them. Parenting your grandchildren not only disrupts your life but deprives the children of grandparents who can spoil them and send them home for their parents to deal with. The children have already lost an important relationship with their parents; now they are losing a precious relationship with you.

Most grandparents, however, don't have other options, and the majority don't want to burden their other adult children. Their only choice is to gear up for the changes and the feelings that come along with raising grandchildren.

▪ *Keep records.* One of the most important things you can do when your grandchildren arrive is to start taking notes. I know that buying notebooks and pens sounds more like preparation for school than for grandparenting, but when you take in your grandchildren, you become more than a surrogate parent; you become their advocate. You may be the only voice speaking solely for their safety and their interests. The law will protect the parents, the government will protect its own pockets, and you will be the one trying to protect your grandchildren's rights—in court, in school, and in the welfare system. You are the one who knows that Dad has a drug problem and that the children are being neglected and/or abused whenever they are with him. You are the one who knows that Max throws tantrums in school after Mom comes to visit. Unfortunately, few people will want to listen to the grandparent, which is why you must document everything. The more organized you are, the better your chances that those who listen will believe you (see Chapter 5).

You will also want to use your notebooks to set yourself up as a kind of central headquarters. Throughout this book you will find lists of the kinds of records you will need to keep: names and phone numbers of attorneys, social workers, and welfare workers connected to your grandchild; the names of their supervisors; and information for school, for doctors, and for the welfare office. The more organized you are from the start, the less crazy you may feel later on.

Remember, the best advocate is an organized one. If you ever need to lock horns with the system, you want to be ready. Keep records of the professionals you talk to and what they tell you. Create a paper trail of letters and documents. Keep dates and times of conversations. Try to write letters when you can and keep copies. Knowledge is power; it may be the only power you have. But nothing you know will do any good if you can't present it in a clear, convincing fashion.

▪ *Sort out the legal maze.* Your grandchildren are family, pure and simple. However, family is also a legal relationship, with rights and responsibilities that can be dictated by the courts. Your rights toward your grandchildren will mostly depend on why they are with you. As soon as possible, find out what your legal rights are in this situation and how you can best protect them. Chapter 10 offers a broad overview of custody issues to get you started, but you will probably want to consult an attorney or other legal professional about your individual case.

▪ *Look into financial aid.* Raising children is expensive. Raising children on a fixed retirement income is expensive and stressful. And raising children on a fixed welfare income, as some grandparents must do, can make you crazy. Whatever obligations you feel you have toward your grandchildren, and I know there are many, you do not have an obligation to support them financally. Financial support is a parent's responsibility. If parents don't fulfill that responsibility, their children are entitled to government assistance.

Many grandparents are reluctant to look to the government for help or don't believe they qualify. They have never asked for help before, and the process mystifies them. Still, while government benefits won't make you rich, every little bit helps, especially Medicaid. As soon as you can, find out what assistance is available to your grandchildren. (For more on government aid, see Chapter 12.)

▪ *Arrange for medical care.* One of the biggest expenses with children is health care. Immunizations and the treatment of colds, earaches, and childhood sprains can add up to a small fortune. Many grandparents are shocked to discover that their insurance companies will not add grandchildren to their policies. However, the children can often be covered by Medicaid. Again, apply early (see Chapter 12).

▪ *Keep medical records.* Accurate medical records can be critical when you raise a child. Few children arrive at grandma's house with records of any kind, but if you can somehow acquire them, they will make your life easier. For instance, have your grandchildren had all their immunization shots? If you don't know, you'll have to start all over. Many grandchildren have had to be reimmunized because of lost records. If the children come to you from a foster care placement or group home, ask the social worker for their medical records. At the very least, try to compile a family medical history based on what you do know about your family. You never know what information could be important later on.

▪ *Enroll them in school.* If you can keep your grandchild in the same school or day-care facility, consider yourself lucky. It's one less change for the child and less stress for you. If not, try to get school records and reports of any special education programs transferred with the child (see Chapter 13). Special education plans should be transferable to the new school, even if it is in another state. Granted, school is much easier to handle in an intact family that was hit by crisis, like a death, than in a family where the parents were on drugs and the child rarely made it to school. Just do the best you can.

▪ *Consider counseling.* Few children are raised by their grandparents for happy reasons. Many grandchildren arrive with emotional, psychological, or behavioral difficulties and/or with physical problems caused by parental abuse or prenatal drug exposure. Most arrive suffering from grief and rejection. If your grandchildren are old enough to talk about feelings and events, consider getting them into counseling. Even if they are too young for counseling on their own, you can work with a counselor on their behalf, learning techniques to help them cope with the situation. I have worked with a number of grandparents to address a child's temper tantrums or inability to sleep in his own bed. These children have all had their lives somehow shattered. A support group or family counseling can start the process of gluing them back together.

▪ *Find your own emotional support.* Raising a second family is stressful and exhausting. It wears on your time, your energy, your finances, and your spirit. Like your grandchildren, you have suffered loss. But you also shoulder the responsibilities. Don't try to do this alone. Look around at your resources. Who can be your emotional support? Whom can you turn to for help? My parents were fortunate. They never worried about baby-sitters because my brother and I were there, although they did worry about burdening us. Many families really are alone. Perhaps your new circumstances involve your only child, or your other children live far away or don't support your taking in the grandchildren. If that is true, you may have to look elsewhere for support. Try other grandparents, a support group, or even a therapist to blow off steam, but do look for help.

CHAPTER 3

Your Lifestyle: Changed and Challenged

It is not the American Dream of a grandparent to raise a second family.
— *Letter from Texas*

Beth Grafton's life was sweet. Her six children were grown, and she was in a wonderful second marriage to Alan, the man of her dreams. Alan had his own business and a comfortable savings. Beth managed a clothing store. If they needed something, they bought it. Alan's father, whom they had nursed for two years, had died the year before, leaving them with the house to themselves and time to rekindle their marriage. After years of renting they were getting ready to buy a home. On weekends Alan would shop and play golf; Beth would do yard work, work on crafts, and visit her grandchildren. In the evenings they would go out to dinner or dancing. Every other month they would join a group of friends in Cape Cod for the weekend.

And they had future plans. They dreamed of taking cruises, since neither one had ever been on one, and of traveling through the United States together. They worried about their adult children but knew they couldn't control their children's lives.

Then the unthinkable happened: Their daughter Ellen was stabbed to death by an abusive husband. To compound the nightmare, the children, who had witnessed the murder, were placed with the father's family, although they had visited their maternal grandparents regularly since they were born and even had their own rooms in their grandparents' house. In addition to the horrible loss of their daughter, Beth and Alan were deprived of seeing their grandchildren.

What followed was three and a half years of court battles that broke the Graftons' bank account and almost broke their spirits. Beth, 51, was described as "an aging, elderly grandmother" and accused of being manic–depressive. "It was as if they were trying to blame Ellen for the murder, and us for raising her that way," says Beth. The Graftons were eventually awarded custody of the children, but the cost of the battle left them shattered. The stress was so high that Alan had three strokes, although a complete physical the year before had judged him to be in great health. He lost his business, and he and Beth spent all their money on attorney fees. Two sons refinanced their own homes to help them out, but Beth and Alan remain thousands of dollars in debt.

Today Beth, Alan, and the children live on Social Security and the money Beth makes from part-time work; she can't find a good full-time job, and they have no medical insurance. In the evenings Beth does laundry, cooks meals, and reads the mail. There are no more dinners out, and the Graftons rarely see their friends, who have different lifestyles.

And their dreams are gone. "I looked forward to when all my kids were gone," says Beth. "I looked forward to being able to find myself as a person, not as a mother or a grandmother but as Beth. It's like I'm lost again, lost raising children. I miss all the things I thought I would be able to do with my husband. All our dreams were ripped out of our book. The whole chapter of our being adults, friends, and lovers together was ripped out, and we're back to raising kids and school and PTA and cookie sales."

LIFESTYLE CHANGES

Raising a child will change your life at any age, but raising a grandchild will turn it upside down. You are no longer young parents with boundless energy; in fact, you might even be at an age when your body betrays you and your health is questionable. You may find yourself in a hornets' nest of social workers and lawyers that nothing has prepared you for. Your own adult child may be your adversary. The system certainly will be. Your routine, your finances, your social life, and your family relationships will all change radically once you have grandchildren under your roof. Your dreams are on hold. Sometimes you might not even recognize the life you are living as your own.

When my mother talks about raising Kevin, her one wish is that she had known other grandparents raising grandchildren, that she had known that what she was going through was normal. Not only are the changes, and the feelings that go with them, normal, but they are almost predictable. Some grandparents have it worse than others, but each one has stories you will probably recognize.

Your Work Life Changes

Alice Brody had been a schoolteacher for 29 years. She hoped to make it to 30 years before she retired. When her daughter's drug addiction left her with the care of several young grandchildren, she had to quit working without reaching her goal. After her daughter died, Ivy Johnson had to go back to work at a grocery store in order to supplement the government assistance she got for her grandchildren. And although Victor Lane had retired at 62, he had to go back to work when he found himself with three new mouths to feed. It's not an easy age to find work, so Victor, a police service officer, works nights and sleeps days, driving 30 miles to and from work each day. One grandfather jokes that he'll be working until he's 90.

Every aspect of work, from a thriving career to a well-earned retirement, can become a casualty of a second parenthood. Child care is expensive, and so is raising children. Some grandparents quit work to save on child care; others return to work to afford the kids. Many trade jobs or rearrange their schedules in an attempt to both work and care for young children. A Pennsylvania grandmother gave up a career in office management to drive a school bus so she could be home when her grandson is home.

You may have to change your work routine. Maybe you worked at night but have to switch to daytime. Will your job be flexible? Will they lay you off? Perhaps you have to reenter the work force. Will you find a job? Can you handle it? The dilemma of working or not working brings up issues of self-esteem and self-worth for many grandparents, as well as the realities of a more modest income and increased stress.

Your Finances Suffer

You worked your whole life and looked forward to your retirement. You may have pensions, social security payments, and savings you had planned to live on. Then your grandchildren arrived. Now you have to use this money for food, clothes, medical bills, and things for the children. "It seems like I can't save anything," says a Michigan grandmother who remembers when she could spend her money freely. "I don't know when I bought my last outfit. Every time I turn around, she is growing."

Court costs can add to the financial stress of raising grandchildren. Some grandparents have sold their homes and watched their nest eggs empty in the fight to get custody of their grandchildren.

If you are a grandparent who has no savings, you face an even greater challenge. It is a severe financial burden to match a lean fixed income with the "unfixed" cost of raising children. Two grandmothers in my GAP groups each have four grandchildren under the age of eight. They live in one-bedroom apartments and can't afford to move in the near future. One can't afford a car; she walks or takes the bus, towing children to school, the doctor, and the market. The other can't even afford a telephone. For grandparents who are also weathering health problems, the lack of a car or telephone can be a catastrophe.

Your Routine Shifts

You had finally adjusted to living without children in the house. You had your own way of doing things, your own schedule. If you put something down, you knew where it was. Your time was yours to work or not work, see friends, read the paper, take leisurely baths, attend to your hobbies. Now your days have been taken over by diapers, bag lunches, and report cards. While your friends are enjoying the company of adults, you are back to the pediatrician, the zoo, and a string of birthday parties. It's tough to keep the house picked up when you have fingerprints and toys scattered everywhere. And your privacy is shot. You have lost your spontaneity to travel or even to eat out. Your day may start at dawn in the rush to tidy the house, cook breakfast, ship the kids off to school, and get to work yourself. For Grandma, it's a distinct feeling of déjà vu. For Grandpa, who may have seen little of his own children while they were growing up, having kids around for 24 hours a day can be quite a shock. For a single grandparent, it's twice as hard.

I received a letter from a teacher in Massachusetts who is raising her three-year-old grandson alone. She finds it difficult to find time for planning her lessons and grading papers, let alone for herself. "I am mother, father, grandparent, and best friend to this little one," she says. "He is not happy to play by himself while I do my school work. I don't think I'd even have time to attend a support group."

No matter how you make your plans, children change your routine. My mother rearranged her work schedule to minimize the disruptions in her grandson's life. Kevin had had to change schools in order to live with my parents after my sister died. Because his life was already falling apart and any consistency was considered important for him, my mother routinely skipped lunch in order to leave work early and pick him up from the same after-school program he had been in before. A New Hampshire grandmother even left her husband back home and spent eight months in Florida so that her granddaughter wouldn't have to switch schools in the middle of the school year. As a grandparent you make many concessions and sacrifices in your routine and lifestyle for the sake of the children.

Your Social Life Declines

"Our circle of friends has dwindled severely because no one else has children," writes a grandmother in Hawaii. "We don't belong with our old friends, nor do we belong with the young parents of our grandchildren's friends," writes another. "I'm a lot older and a lot wiser parent this time," says a third. "But with the Brownies, the gymnastics, the parents' nights, and the sudden earaches, we've lost our entire circle of friends. Our lives are on hold, indefinitely."[1]

It is a complaint that many grandparents recognize: Your social life and your hobbies decrease when the grandchildren arrive. Longtime friends are caught up with activities they couldn't do when they were raising families; they don't want kids tagging along. Perhaps you live in an older neighborhood with few children. Your friends may no longer have childproof homes. "Our friends raised their kids," says one grandmother. "They don't want hyperactive children in their homes."[2] Even when you can get together with friends your own age, the cost of baby-sitting is one more expense on an already stretched budget.

Single grandparents, particularly single grandmothers, may also struggle with issues of romantic companionship. Many children try to interfere with these relationships. Children may be insecure about a male friend getting Grandma's attention because her dating may bring back memories of their mother's giving more attention to men than to them. One 43-year-old woman who is raising her ex-husband's grandchildren wrote, "My life is on hold because I am never going to find a husband or have a life of my own till they are grown, and by then I will be well into my 60s."

Your Dreams Disappear

More than your immediate lifestyle changes when the second shift arrives; your future changes, too. Plans get put on hold, and some dreams disappear altogether. It's another loss in a long line of losses. Jack and Betty Segal had plans for this time of their lives. Jack would be retired and they would be out on the road together some-where—alone. Instead, they are raising one child of a drug-addicted son and helping a divorced daughter raise three more. "You love the kids," says Betty. "You just resent the fact that you can't be doing what you want to be doing."

Emily Petersen didn't have big plans. She's a quiet person who had looked forward to a tidy home, solitary walks, and presiding over holiday dinners like a traditional grandma. Instead, she is surrogate mother to an active grandchild and can hardly find a minute for herself.

"We planned retirement to do what we wanted to do; it was our time in life," one grandmother told a reporter. "Now we can't even watch the evening news because that's cartoon time."[3] Resentment. It isn't a word we traditionally associate with grandchildren. But when your life changes so radically, it unleashes a torrent of complex and contradictory emotions.

AN EMOTIONAL ROLLER COASTER

As soon as Karlos Gregory heard her grandson was coming, she got in gear: She found a day-care center, talked to an attorney about custody, and turned one room into a little boy's bedroom. When he arrived, she washed his clothes, bought new tennis shoes, and brought a night-light down from the attic. But she wasn't prepared for the feelings that come with the new responsibility and the loss of freedom. "At age 54, all of a sudden I've got a 4-year-old. Nobody seems to understand where I'm coming from," she told a local reporter.[4]

Every grandparent I know would understand. On any given day they can go through a full spectrum of feelings: grief and shame for their grown children, love for their grandchildren, fear for a future in which their health and finances may dwindle, resentment at a juvenile court system that treats them with disrespect, anger at losing their dreams at this time of their lives, and guilt for feeling that anger. The rapid shifts of emotion are like a roller coaster. Your life is in constant turmoil. Of course you feel unstable.

How much these feelings shake you will depend on what kind of resources and support you have. A single grandparent has a tougher time dealing with the ups and downs of second parenthood than a married couple, who can rely on each other to shoulder some of the weight. Two people may not reach their wit's end at the same time; a single grandparent may have no one else to turn to. Either way, it is important to look at these feelings, to really feel them, to give yourself time to deal with the issues they represent. The more you bury feelings, the more likely they are to fester inside you, erupting like a volcano when you least expect it. "It seems to take about a year to stop denying that this unexpected role is not a temporary situation," writes a grandmother from Oklahoma. "From my standpoint, we all need to know and understand that the cycle of shock, resentment, loneliness, guilt and, finally, acceptance is perfectly normal."

Isolation

If there is one theme that runs through every letter and phone call I receive from grandparents, it is isolation. When you parent for the second time, it is a lonely feeling. You feel like you're the only one in the world in this situation. You don't fit in with young parents at school functions, but you don't feel right taking small children to seniors' events. "My husband and I have permanent custody of a four-year-old grandson and find ourselves outcasts in most settings, including visits to the pediatrician," writes one grandmother.

You may also feel alienated from your family and friends. Of course you feel isolated. You *are* isolated. Your world turned upside down, and not many people can accept your new role. Loneliness and even depression are normal, expected reactions to all this over-whelming change. Seek out others who understand, either in a one-on-one relationship or through a support group. It sounds simple, but it's true: The best antidote to isolation is other people.

Grief

Every grandparent raising a grandchild experiences many losses, as well as the deep grief that comes with them. In some cases it is the death of your own child, your grandchild's parent. Your grandchild is a constant reminder of that loss. One grandfather says that the sight of his grandchild always reminds him that his son is dead. "It's a painful thing to live with," he says. In other cases the parent can't parent. This brings a different kind of grief. This adult is not the child you raised. You have lost the bright child with unlimited potential; you have lost the faith that your child would someday be a good parent and a productive adult.

In a sense, you also lose the special relationship with your grand-children that makes grandparenting so wonderful: the visits, the spoil-ing, the special treats, the grandparent–grandchild conspiracies. You may feel cheated out of your grandparent role and mourn its loss.

Grandparents whose adult children have died can find solid sup-port and understanding through Compassionate Friends, a national organization for parents who have lost a child. We have also had grandparents and grandchildren benefit from counseling or from be-reavement groups, that is, short-term counseling groups that deal specifically with the phases of loss and how to deal with grief. Ask your local hospital or hospice for a referral; social workers, attorneys, doctors, and senior centers may also keep referral lists. Understand that anniversaries and holidays will be emotional times for you, and be on guard against plummeting depression. You need time to grieve, and it is understandable that you might want to grieve in private. However, some people progressively isolate themselves under the weight of depression, and then they can't pull themselves back up. If you can't reach out to people, at least don't push them away. You need loving support to withstand this loss.

It is almost easier to discuss grief when an adult child has died. Grandparents who have lost a child to drugs or mental illness yo-yo back and forth from grief to hope and back again. Here, too, support groups are helpful. Even if your child is living, allow yourself to grieve. Make room for it. You too are suffering severe loss—the loss of your dreams for your adult child, of your relationship with that child, of your lifestyle, and of your grandparent role.

Anger and Guilt

Anger and guilt are familiar companions to many second-time parents. Anger at fate. Anger at the courts and the bureaucracy, which make you feel victimized and penalized for taking responsibility for your grandchildren, especially when you have exhausted your savings and your energy. Anger at your adult child for putting you in this situation. "I could beat that woman for days for what she did to that baby!" said Anne Sutter, whose daughter gave birth to a drug-exposed child and then abandoned him.

You may even get angry at your grandchildren, who are the real victims but who are also the ones who have changed your life. Even when you know that it is not the children's fault, you may still feel resentment—and then guilt for feeling it. "You feel this hostility," says Fay Strassburger. "You feel this frustration. You lose your identity. What are you going to do with these kids? And, then, when they look up at you, you say, 'God, just let me get through another day because they really need me.'"[5]

Lucy Davis is raising her son's daughter, Lindsey. Her son and his girlfriend were both teenagers and drug addicts when Lindsey was born. Lucy took the baby when the mother lost custody for child abuse. Like many grandparents, she thought this would be temporary; she thought that losing custody would scare the parents into shape and that her own life would go back to normal. When that didn't happen, she adopted the child. She loves her completely, but sometimes the frustration is overwhelming: "I should just have to come home and make my bed, and the house should look the way I left it. But it doesn't. There are Barbie dolls everywhere. There's a toy room to be picked up. There's all her laundry to be done. Her dentist appointments. Her eye appointments. She takes up a tremendous part of my time. You can't just call me for drinks; I have

Lindsey. I get angry about it inside, although I don't want to show it. But then when she comes in and breaks a lamp, I'm really angry. And I feel so guilty."

It is okay to feel angry. Your life has been disrupted, and it is normal to resent it. What you don't want to do is take out those feelings on your grandchild. One way to defuse your anger is to write it down. Keep a journal or diary, or write a letter to the child's parents—even if you can't (or wouldn't) send it. Just getting your feelings out on paper can help. Find people who can be a sounding board for your feelings. But don't wait for a crisis to call them; call *before* you reach the end of your rope.

Fear

Grandparents who parent live in a kind of low-grade constant fear, haunted by the courts, the parents, their own health issues, and the steady march of time. Not only are they struggling with severe changes to their lives, but they are often battling the normal aging process, if not illnesses like diabetes, arthritis, cataracts, heart problems, and cancer. The questions buzz around them like mosquitos: "What if something happens to me? Who will raise these children?" "What if the parents resurface?" "What if the system lets the parents take the kids before they are able to care for them?" "How will my grandchildren turn out?" "What effect will all this have on them?"

The hard part about these fears is that they are real and possible. Parents do resurface. Courts do give them priority. Grandparents do get sick and die. And the reality is that many of these children could end up in foster care, separated from siblings, despite every effort to keep them together. A grandmother in one of my GAP groups died of breast cancer this year. Now the family is struggling over her two grandchildren; her other children don't want them, and their mother is still on drugs.

There is not much you can do about these fears. You have to look at them head-on. It doesn't help to put them aside to deal with later—although you may do that for a while. Eventually, however, you need to plan for what you can affect and, as painful as it is, accept what you cannot change. You can, and should, make decisions about who takes the children if something happens to you. If you don't have custody, there really isn't anything you can do if the parents resurface. But living in fear won't prevent it from happening. Although you can't erase your fears, try not to let them overwhelm you.

Doubt

Emily Petersen sometimes wonders if she did the right thing by taking her granddaughter Amanda, if she would have been better off adopted by younger parents. "Maybe we drown in the love for the child—the fear for the child—that we don't stop to think that maybe a younger family, someone a little more prosperous, might give them a better life," she says, pointing out that as older grandparents she and Carter are often not able to do for Amanda what they would like to do. "Some days I get terribly tired," she says.

Doubt, for many grandparents, is a normal part of raising grandchildren. You think it's not fair to the kids that you can't play ball or roller-skate or do many of the things you did as young parents. You do get tired and stressed. But I feel that in most cases children are still better off with family, if the family is able to provide for them. Whether you have made the best choice for yourself, however, is something only you can know.

▪ HOW TO COPE

There is no question that your grandchildren have brought incredible change and challenge into your life. How you approach these changes, and the feelings that accompany them, will determine how well an adjustment is made by everyone involved. As you move into a life with your grandchild, here are a few key points to remember:

▪ *Prioritize.* Decide what is most important and handle that first. Do you need to get back to work to pay bills? Then child care is primary. Don't worry about summer child care if it's just January; think about after-school care.

▪ *Don't just take one day at a time; take one thing at a time.* Get the children ready for school, then make your shopping list and schedule your afternoon. Plan for small increments.

▪ *Take time for yourself.* Structure your life in a way that works for you; find a routine that gives you downtime. What gives you a little bit of pleasure? What can you do to refuel? Is it a movie? Reading the paper? Make time for it. When you are constantly giving, giving, giving, you aren't taking care of yourself. And if you fall apart, physically or emotionally, there will be no one to take care of those grandchildren, and they could end up in foster care. So treat yourself regularly, even if it is just a quiet bath.

▪ *Make life easy.* You don't have to cook full meals every night. You don't have to have a perfect home. Try lowering your standards and lightening your load. It's okay to pop frozen food in the microwave. It's okay to go out for fast food. This is about emotional survival.

▪ *Set limits with your grandchildren.* You will have less resentment about sacrificing your life if you don't give up every aspect of it. Setting rules and limits, like private time or a regular bedtime (earlier than yours!), will give you a little time here and there for yourself.

▪ *Ask for help.* Look for *people* support. If you have supportive friends, use them. Also, find other people who have gone through what you are going through. Check with a senior citizens' group, or ask your grandchild's teacher and pediatrician if they know other people in the same situation. It's important to know you're not alone.

▪ *Get into a support group.* Therapy and support groups are a safe second family. You will be able to talk about your feelings without being judged or criticized. Other grandparents may be able to help you prioritize when you just can't think anymore. You may also find resources in a group: a clothing exchange, grandparents who might be home in the afternoon and willing to watch a child for a few hours. Grandparents who have been in the group for a while are often more than willing to give back to someone in a worse predicament. The fewer resources you have on hand, the more you need to seek outside support. Even if you are well connected in a community, with lots of friends, you can benefit from a support group. The majority of your friends are probably not in the same situation.

▪ *Consider your religious community.* Many people get strength from their faith. I know a number of grandparents who say that prayer and the support of their church or synagogue can help immensely. Some congregations have even provided material support to grandparents in emergency situations.

▪ *Let yourself off the hook.* You need to accept the fact that your adult child's circumstances are not your fault. Your child is making choices, and you have done the most and best with whatever you had. I don't think people intentionally set out to hurt their kids, and when you raised yours, you really thought what you were doing was the best. Understand that your feelings are normal, that you're not alone, and that you will eventually get through this.

▪ *Focus on the positive.* Keep in mind why you are doing this and what you have accomplished. In spite of all the stress, there are rewards.

MOMENTS OF PURE JOY

Grandparents sacrifice a lot to raise grandchildren, but there are rewards: the relief of knowing that the grandchildren are safe and happy, the wonder of watching them grow, the pride in their accomplishments. Some grandparents say their grandchildren keep them young. Alta Edwards believes her three grandchildren gave her a new lease on life. She had diabetes, arthritis, a bad heart, and high blood pressure, and she weighed 300 pounds. "One morning I woke up and realized I couldn't properly raise a two-year-old flat on my back. It was do or die," she says. "They got me back on my feet."[6]

And there is the love. It is the main reason you took in your grandchildren, and it is your greatest reward for raising them. "Nobody has ever loved me in my life the way she loves me," says Lucy Davis of her granddaughter. "She was singing a song one day, when she was three. She was in her toy room, and she was singing, 'I have a mummy and her name is Grammy!'"

Joan McMillin knows the feeling. She remembers the night her granddaughter hugged her and said, "Granny, you're the only person in the world who really loves me." "I had tears in my eyes," she told a reporter. "There's something positively magical in the hugs and kisses that makes it all worthwhile."[7]

CHAPTER 4

Family at Large: Your Spouse and Other Children

> You're going to be fighting the battle alone at times. Your friends, even your family, will fight you for raising grandchildren. They each have their own version of how you should handle the situation, and you have to face their advice and their criticism.
>
> —*Vermont grandmother*

T aking in a grandchild is about family, and the entire family will feel the effects of this new addition. More than your lifestyle changes when you become second-time parents; your marriage and your relationship with your other children may suffer strains you never expected.

ROCKING THE MARRIAGE BOAT

Ivy Johnson's husband left her when the grandchildren arrived. Frank and Gloria Simon fight constantly over their drug-addicted daughter. And my own parents seemed close to divorce on numerous occasions. The burden of raising a child at this stage of life, combined with the loss of or struggles with an adult child (regardless of the reason), often causes deep problems between spouses who have spent most of their lives together. Marriages that have always been stable start to develop rifts, and marriages that were already strained may split wide open.

Sometimes the issue is grief. Everyone grieves differently, and you expect different things of each other in your grief. My parents didn't have time to mourn the loss of my sister before they took in her son. My mother expressed it all openly: She cried constantly and all but lived at the cemetery when she wasn't working. My father, on the other hand, buried his grief deep inside himself, and my mother would get furious at his apparent lack of understanding. Grief can rock the most stable marriage, even without the extra burden of new children to raise.

Sometimes the issue is jealousy: One grandparent gives more attention to the child than to his or her spouse, who resents the change and may then spend more time away from home, become engrossed in hobbies, or generally keep the family at a distance. Growing anger may spark fights and arguments over seemingly meaningless things. Often it is Grandma who devotes herself to the grandchildren and Grandpa who rebels. Says one grandfather from Ohio, "We get along, no fights, no shouting matches . . . but [the child] has caused a deterioration of our compatibility . . . I feel pretty much ignored."[1]

But grandmothers are not immune from jealousy, as Nancy Harper can confirm. "He probably loves her more than me," she says, referring to her husband and the granddaughter they are raising. "My husband was such a wonderful father, and everything was 'the children.' I thought once they grew up I'd have him all to myself. Then Scott presented us with Marissa, and here we are all over again."

The sudden changes to your lifestyle will certainly challenge a marriage. Financial stress is always hard on a couple, and unexpected children's expenses raise new questions about how to spend money and how to set priorities. Adjustments to work and home routines leave you with little time for yourself, for each other, for all the things you planned. And then there is the disruption to your privacy and sexual intimacy.

Rose and Gerald Avery had been married for 30 years. Ever since their son Richard moved out, they had been peacefully on their own. At the end of a long day their house was a haven of quiet, order, and privacy. They liked it that way. They could walk around the house wearing anything they wanted to; they could be intimate and sexual without fear of being heard. When they welcomed Richard and his two young sons into their home, that peace and privacy disappeared. At the end of the day the house is now riddled with the sounds and signs of children: laughter, arguments, toys on the floor. Gerald's office is now the television room. Even their bedroom isn't their own—the boys always want to be with them. Their new circumstances have taken a toll on the couple's intimacy. Even when the children aren't home, they live with the expectation that they could come home at any moment. "At times, it's like we've lost the house and certain things about each other," says Rose. The result is that Gerald is often angry. "It's like having four kids at home, not two," she adds.

The most constant source of marital conflict, however, is the children—both the adult children and the grandchildren. In both cases the issues are overcompensation and setting limits. Each is a normal issue in childrearing, but having to negotiate these boundaries at a stage in your life when you no longer expect to be rearing your child and expect only to be enjoying your grandchild can wear on you and your marriage.

Children, Big and Small

Many couples can't agree as to when enough is enough when it comes to their adult children. Whether the issue is money, visitation, or kicking them out, they are incapable of presenting a united front. One grandparent tries to take a firm stand and the other undermines it. One grandparent feels misunderstood, the other unsupported. If the conflict escalates enough, talk can turn to separation and divorce. That is what almost happened to Frank and Gloria Simon.

Frank and Gloria took in their grandchildren when their oldest daughter, Cheryl, divorced her abusive husband and lost custody of her little girls because of drug abuse and neglect. When I met this family, Cheryl was living at home again, sleeping all day and making Gloria's life miserable. She was verbally abusive to her children and to her mother in front of the children. She felt that her mother had stolen her daughters. When she was under the influence of drugs, Cheryl became violent: She pulled Gloria's hair, threw her to the ground, knocked out windows. But Frank kept supporting Cheryl, and it took forever for Gloria to put her out of the house.

Frank refused to believe the severity of the problem. He worked all day and wasn't home to witness what his daughter was doing. Besides, Cheryl was "Daddy's little girl," and he wanted to believe everything would work out. He gave her chance after chance, undermining his wife: Gloria would reach a breaking point and tell Cheryl she couldn't stay with them, and Frank would let her back in. Or

Cheryl would break a window to come into the house, and Frank would let her stay. He refused to back Gloria on setting limits of any kind, whether expressed verbally or in written contracts.

The Simons' marriage almost collapsed under the strain. When things were particularly bad, Gloria would pile the children into the car and call me from a pay phone. "I can't stand it anymore," she would say, sobbing. "I'm running away and leaving Frank." She always returned home, but she was stuck in a tough situation. As long as the Simons weren't working together, nothing could change. Then one day Frank himself became the target of Cheryl's anger. It was only when his daughter threw a toaster and hit him in the head that Frank put his foot down and joined Gloria in her insistence that Cheryl move out of their home.

When it comes to the *grandchildren*, two problems typically shake a relationship: first whether to take the children, and then how to raise them. Sometimes a grandmother will leave a marriage to be able to take in and protect a small grandchild. Sometimes a grandfather will leave when the children arrive. Writes a woman from Arizona: "I'm 59 and raised seven of my own children and three grandchildren. My husband left me over this last child after 33 years of marriage, but I can't seem to let [this grandchild] go." Emily and Carter Petersen had their marriage pulled almost to the breaking point when their daughter asked them to take her child. Emily and Carter were already raising their son's baby, and Carter didn't want any more. They got into a huge fight about it. "I told him if we can't take care of two, we're not taking care of one," recalls Emily. "If I can care for another girl's baby, I can certainly take care of my daughter's. If you don't like it, you go," she told him. "But the baby's coming in." Faced with that choice, Carter stayed.

The day-to-day task of raising grandchildren is more of a slow wear and tear on a marriage. One grandparent tries to parent, with all the struggle, limit setting, and discipline that parenting entails. Meanwhile, the other one overcompensates for the child's lack of parents and tries to hang on to the role of the sweet, loving grandparent. The result is strife for the grandparents and confused signals for the child.

My parents fought constantly over Kevin, who was not an easy child to raise. My mother overcompensated, giving in to many of Kevin's demands. My father criticized how she handled the child, but he traveled for business and wasn't often there to help. They felt anger and grief; they fought and screamed. Even homework was a horrible scene. Every night for months my brother and I would take turns dropping in to check on them and to smooth things over.

It's true that every couple has its fights and bones of contention, but by the time you are grandparents you don't expect to be arguing about small children. You don't expect to be fighting about your grandchildren: you expect to be loving them, doting on them, and sending them home. In grandparenting you have regressed, and there is an added layer of frustration about the change. To quote one grandmother: "Fifty percent of my anxiety and stress is the old boy [Grandpa]. He fights everything I do."

Strength in a Common Cause

Not every marriage suffers from the arrival of grandchildren. There are couples who find that the challenge of raising a second family draws them together instead of pulling them apart.

Dave and Milly Walsh are raising four grandchildren, and their disruptive daughter is still in and out of the house. Dave works nights, Milly is at home with the children, and the daughter doesn't contribute a dime. Milly's health isn't great. The couple would love to travel alone for once, just the two of them, but it's not likely to happen soon. They're both exhausted. It's fertile soil for conflict, but they don't feel it. "Our marriage is not a flashy thing," says Milly. "It keeps going on." Humor and a strong sense of purpose keep them going. Says Dave, "Every six months we think, 'What are we doing? We're supposed to be retired!' But we laugh at each other when we're blue. We want to be doing what we're doing. It's not duty; we're bonded to these kids. If anything, it made us stronger. We're doing something together. People tend to drift apart as they get older; we have a common cause. We're channeling our energy into something constructive."

■ HOW TO COPE

How well your marriage survives will depend on how stable it is to start with, how much stress you have to handle, and how committed you and your spouse are to surviving as a couple. The road will be easier, however, if you keep certain things in mind:

▪ *Talk to each other!* Often, when couples disagree, they shut down and withdraw; then they aren't open to compromise and discussion. Taking on your grandchildren will add new dimensions of stress to your marriage; try to keep the paths of communication open.

▪ *Create special time for yourself and your spouse.* It is critical that grandparents take time away from the grandchildren; you need this to refuel yourselves and your relationship. You are both losing out on your plans and dreams for this time together. You must make a conscious effort to do things that make you feel good, or they just won't happen. I know it is hard to plan your own activities when you're overwhelmed by three or four needy, active kids; it's hard to think about yourself when you are so exhausted that you collapse in bed at night and hope you don't have to get up. But you have to make the effort. Your health, your sanity, and your marriage could depend on it.

▪ *Present a unified front to your grandchildren.* It is important not to argue or contradict each other in front of the grandchildren because (1) they already have low self-esteem and feel that everything is their fault and (2) they can manipulate your disagreement to their advantage (children are good at pitting one grandparent against the other to get what they want). When there is an issue to deal with, try to discuss it beforehand, or take a time-out to discuss it. If you are split in your decision, your grandchild may try to play you against each other, which helps neither your decision making nor your relationship.

▪ *Present a united front to your adult children, too.* They are expert manipulators and know which of you to go to when they want something. Discuss limits and boundaries in advance and then stick to them. (For more on adult children, see Chapter 5.)

▪ *Try to keep things in perspective.* It won't make the situation easier, but it can preserve your sense of humor. It also helps when you can lean on each other for support.

SIBLING SUPPORT AND SIBLING RIVALRY: YOUR OTHER CHILDREN

Grace and Marcus Tyler have three grown children. Their only daughter lost custody of her five-year-old son, Jason, because of drugs and neglect, and now they are raising him. Their son Michael, 29, lives out of town with his girlfriend and his daughter. He doesn't see his parents or his nephew often, but he supports their decision to raise Jason. He calls often and takes the boy for occasional weekends. The Tylers' other son, Peter, 25, lives only a few blocks away. In the past, if he didn't see his parents every week, he would at least call two or three times to touch base with them. Now he rarely comes around at all. He says he will help with Jason, but he never does. Moreover, he complains to his brother about their parents' devotion to Jason: "Do you think they would take care of our kids that well? Look at all the attention he's getting. He's spoiled rotten!" "Peter has been jealous from the moment that Jason came into the house," says Grace. "You'd think that he would understand that this is an innocent child who deserves a chance. What are we taking away from a 25-year-old man?"

Two sons, two reactions, and there is nothing surprising about either one. Many lives are touched when a grandchild moves in, and many relationships are disrupted. The other children in your family are not immune to the situation. If they live with you or near you, they may find their own lives altered. Even if they live far away, they may be rocked by unexpected emotions due to this new arrangement. They may be jealous of the drain on your time and attention. They may be afraid of the toll on your health and your marriage. And they may be furious with their sibling for "taking advantage of Mom and Dad." They may even be angry at you for, in their eyes, allowing yourself to be taken advantage of. Some, like Michael, may offer to help out; some may punish you by withholding their support; and others may simply ignore the whole situation, keeping a polite but neutral distance. How your other children choose to handle their feelings will depend on their ages, their circumstances, and their prior relationships with you.

Other Children at Home

Joyce Griffin's children were in their teens when, one at a time, the grandchildren started coming—all from one daughter and all drug exposed. Joyce had already raised five children and had nursed two husbands through injuries and disease. Her other children were not pleased with this new turn of events. "My children thought I was deserving of rest," she says. "They didn't see me starting over raising children, especially drug children." So when the fourth call came, Joyce's oldest son said, "No more." Then he saw the baby, who had been born five weeks early. "When they saw the preemie—how small, how vulnerable she was—then my children became mothers and fathers," says Joyce. "My sons became the fathers to these children; my younger daughter, who is in college, became the mother."

Nancy Harper's daughter, Jennifer, was 16 when little Marissa arrived. Her brother Scott, the baby's father, was 18, and her oldest brother was 22. Jennifer had been the only girl in the family, the light of her mother's life. The baby's arrival was hard for her. Not only was there competition from a needy child in the house, but it seemed as if her life had been taken away: She couldn't run her blow-dryer at night because the baby was sleeping, and she found herself watching her brother's baby daughter while Scott disappeared with his friends. Jennifer was angry at everyone involved. When Nancy asked her to take Marissa for a few hours, her response was, "Why should I, Mom? I'm going out with friends. I didn't have a baby, Scott did. Just because your life stinks, mine won't, too."

Children who still live at home will, of course, be most affected by a grandchild moving in. Like you, they will find their routine and their living space disrupted by the new addition to the family. They may be asked to share their rooms, to limit their activities, and, if they're old enough, to watch a niece or nephew when you need a break. Unlike you, they had no choice in the matter. From their perspective, a new child arrived and began to take over. A child living at home may feel lost amid all these changes. If, like Jennifer, the child has been the baby of the family, she may feel displaced by this new arrival. Younger children may act out to get more of your time and attention, and even young adults may experience jealousy.

Sometimes feelings of jealousy in your children predate your grandchild's arrival. Marlena Hunt's younger daughter already felt ignored growing up, mostly because she was the "good" kid and Marlena was so caught up with her sister Sharon and her problems. Now Marlena is giving her attention to Sharon's daughter.

Of course, the moments of competition and resentment may be much more sporadic once the novelty passes and everyone settles into a new routine. But when you raise a grandchild as one of your own children, you will always get some sibling rivalry.

When Siblings Are Single Adults

Sandra Cobb has two sons and two daughters. She is raising seven grandchildren while their mother is in and out of jail and rehab. Both her sons have been helpful, but her daughter JoAnne has been her right hand. She was 16 when the babies started to arrive, and has been like another mother to them, even though the wear and tear on her 65-year-old mother makes her angry. Although JoAnne now has children of her own, she still lives next door and helps out with her nieces and nephews.

My parents were equally lucky. My brother and I were both single adults when my sister died. We had no commitments, no children, and we were already close to our nephew. Like Joyce Griffin's children, Phil and I pitched in, becoming extra parents to Kevin and taking some of the pressure off our parents. No decision was made without us, and Kevin even lived with each of us at one point or another. Even so, we recognized the differences between the way our parents raised Kevin and the way they raised us. We watched our mother overcompensate, and we watched Kevin get away with things that we would never have gotten away with as children. Phil and I would voice our disapproval and offer suggestions, but these were frequently ignored because my parents thought they were doing the right thing.

Single adults who don't live at home may be less personally affected by your decision to raise a grandchild. Whether they approve of the decision or not, they have the freedom to make their own choices about being involved. Some might even become active aunts and uncles, as JoAnne, Phil, and I did, possibly challenging some parenting techniques, but steadily helping with day care and vacations and acting as parental stand-ins when needed. (My brother even coached Kevin's Little League team.)

Other single adult children, like Grace Tyler's son Peter, may be actively *un*involved. They may vocally disapprove of your choice and may take it out on you by distancing themselves. They may ignore their niece or nephew, neglecting to ask about the child or even send a birthday card. Some may genuinely feel displaced and hurt by the time and attention showered on your grandchild. "But they are adults!" you say in wonder. Yes, but they are still your children.

Many single adults are neither active aunts and uncles nor active critics. These are the neutral ones. They may be caught up with their own lives. They may live far away. They just aren't involved.

When Siblings Are Married with Children

The reactions of married adult children are not very different from those of single adults unless there are other grandchildren in the picture. Then you risk a new kind of sibling rivalry: cousin rivalry.

> "You spend so much energy on Marcia that my kids never see you!"
> "You do so much more for Martin's kids than you ever do for mine."
> "Grandma, how come you buy so many things for Tommy? Don't you love me, too?"

These are the complaints that can break a grandparent's heart. It is hard enough when they come from small grandchildren who don't really understand the situation, but it can be incredibly frustrating when they come from an adult who knows that Marcia, Tommy, and Martin's kids have no one else spending time and money on them. It is particularly painful when, deep down, you know the accusations are true. And it's not fair.

Sue Ellen Rice would love to indulge all her grandchildren, but she is raising two little ones on a meager income. The rest live several states away, and she can't afford to visit them; she can't even afford to send much in the way of presents. It doesn't make her feel like much of a grandma. Ethel Murray's problem is closer to home. Scott, the grandson she is raising, is the same age as his cousin, Aaron, who lives down the street. Aaron sees that Scott gets special things and thinks that Grandma loves him more. Aaron's mother adds to Ethel's guilt with her own complaints. Ethel has explained to Aaron that he has a mommy to buy him things and Scott doesn't. Although she tries to pick up special things for Aaron when she can, the competition between the cousins still disturbs her.

On the other hand, not every married adult child will resent the time and attention spent on a sibling's child. Some will go out of their way to be supportive, including the child in their own family activities and vacations. Sometimes the same sibling who opposed your grand-child's arrival may, like Joyce Griffin's son, become a doting surrogate parent over time. It all depends on the particular relationships in your family.

Remember Nancy Harper's teenage daughter? Jennifer didn't even want to babysit Marissa, but when Jennifer reached adulthood and married, she and her husband offered to lighten Nancy's responsi-bilities and raise the little girl themselves. Nancy declined. "Marissa has already felt rejection once," she explains. "She's already had one mummy leave her, and this mummy's not going to." Still, Jennifer had made the offer.

▪ HOW TO COPE

The preceding vignettes illustrate just a few of the reactions your other children could have to your raising a grandchild. You may find yourself facing completely different ones, depending on your particular circumstances and your relationships with your children. Moreover, each of your children will have his own individual approach to handling the feelings involved. However they react, there are a few things you may want to consider in dealing with your other children and as a means of keeping peace in your family:

▪ *Listen to your other children.* They deserve to have their con-cerns heard. First of all, their concerns may be valid. Perhaps you *are* overcompensating with your grandchild; you may be hurting her in the process. Perhaps you are neglecting your teenagers; maybe you can arrange some special time together. See if you can find a compromise without sacrificing yourself. Second, the feelings of your other children are valid even if you can't do anything about their concerns. You may not be able to buy *all* your grandchildren new shoes, but you can try to understand how your other children and grandchildren might feel slighted, however illogical their reaction may seem.

▪ *Validate their feelings.* Everyone reacts differently to crisis, and having your family structure upset is a kind of crisis. It doesn't matter whether your other children are feeling scared about your health, jealous of your time, or sorry for the grandchild you are raising. They are entitled to their feelings, and those feelings are normal. All you can do is try to understand and not take it too personally. You do not, however, have to let them take their disapproval out on you.

▪ *Don't expect their help.* In your heart you will want the support and assistance of your other children. You can let them know you would appreciate it, but don't expect anything from them. They have a right to their own opinions about the situation, and they have to make their own decisions about how they want to participate. Besides, wouldn't you rather have them help because they want to help?

The situation is different when your other children live at home. It is reasonable to have certain expectations of children who live under your roof. Perhaps everyone in your house shares chores and responsibilities; child care may now be one of those responsibilities. However, try to be sensitive to the needs of your children. You don't want to deprive them of time to do their homework or see their friends

▪ *Consider instituting family meetings.* It is easy for members of a family to retire to their own respective corners to nurse their injuries and strengthen their opinions; you could end up as a group of disconnected loners instead of an integrated family. Whether your other children live at home or not, the family meeting can be a way of keeping everyone connected. If your other children feel neglected, you can invite them to participate in certain decisions. If they feel taken advantage of, they can air out their concerns. I can't overemphasize how important communication is in a family, particularly in times of stress.

▪ *Don't forget your other grandchildren.* It doesn't take much time or money to make a child feel remembered, even in another state. Sometimes just a postcard is enough. Be patient if the other grandchildren need repeated explanations about why Tommy gets more toys. It will take them a while to adjust to the situation, too.

▪ *Make your own decisions.* It is good to listen to your other adult children and to recognize their concerns, but in the end you have to follow your conscience, particularly when it comes to taking your grandchild. The bottom line is that when the day is over and the lights go out, the decisions you make have to be the ones you can sleep with.

Remember, there are no perfect families, only people who are striving.

CHAPTER 5

Your Adult Child

My son has destroyed all of us and is continuing
to do so. We just cannot get rid of him. He is
just a shell of a person we loved so much. The
hurt is in me so deep, and I always ask why.
—*Letter from Missouri*

S he was a beautiful, bright, and gifted child,
the oldest of my three children," writes Pam
Marshall. "She was reliable, sensitive, and
unusually creative. During her grade school years, she never gave
us any trouble. She studied hard. She helped her younger sister and
brother with their homework. Teachers all loved her. In junior high
she started to change." Pam is describing her daughter Linda, and at
first it sounds like a typical 1960s story of teenage rebellion—flower
children, hard rock, heavy makeup and miniskirts, a little marijuana,
moving out of the house—the kind of thing a lot of adults today
experienced, and outgrew.

But Linda didn't outgrow it. By age 19, she was using heroin.
When her parents offered to get her help, she told them her friends
were her family now and walked out of the house. Heroin was re-
placed by LSD, uppers, downers, cocaine, and crack—anything she
could get her hands on. Linda got married twice and divorced twice.
She was arrested several times on drug-related charges. At 32 she
gave birth to a baby girl in jail. Pam and her husband, Robert, took
the infant home from the hospital and have raised her ever since.

Linda's story is not an unusual one. In fact, it is all too usual.
It is the story of the troubled adult child, the parent of the child you

are raising, the author of the situation you are in. No discussion of grandparents as parents is complete without looking at the adult who is still in the picture.

It is a sad fact, but grandparents who are raising the children of dead or absent parents have a much simpler time of it. Except for the cases—and there are some—where grandparents raise grandchildren in cooperation with the parents, adult children seem to have one mission in life: wreaking havoc in your life. For many families it is not the grandchild who is the problem, it is the parent.

A PICTURE OF THE ADULT CHILD

Among the letters I have received is one from a young woman in New York. The picture she paints is a common one: Her mother, a woman in her early 50s, is raising her sister's two toddlers. The sister lives with the mother but doesn't help with the children. She spends any money she has on herself—on drugs, clothing, jewelry, and the boyfriend of the week. She disappears for days at a time, returning only to pick up her welfare check. "My sister has taken the car and told my mom she's going to the grocery store and doesn't come back for a week," the young woman writes. "My sister abandoned the kids one night to go out with friends." The grandmother has bruises from the children's mother, and her jewelry is gone. She needs financial assistance and custody of the children. She needs to get her daughter out of her house, but she is afraid for the safety of the babies.

Some grandparents call them "deadbeat" moms and dads. These are the parents who show up long enough to make promises, break promises, and disappear again. At best, these parents occasionally visit and indulge their children while you and your spouse play Mom and Dad. Linda brings her daughter presents and tries to be a model mother, but her interest doesn't last long. "My daughter loves her daughter," says Pam. "She wants to hold her, dress her up, play with her . . . like a traditional grandparent who comes for two hours." At worst, they can be verbally and physically abusive to you and their children. I heard from Michigan grandparents who took their grandchildren when one of the men the mother lived with, an ex-convict, was preparing a tattoo for their grandson. Because the mother was overheard threatening to blow up the grandparents' car and apartment, the family fled to another state, from which they notified the authorities that they had left, and why.

Many adult children are manipulative. They may use their children as pawns to extort money, shelter, and transportation from you. And if you have no legal control over your grandchildren, you will probably give in. Grandparents are the first to admit that they have bought more drugs than any other class of people by giving into their adult children's demands in order to protect their grandchildren.

Your adult child may also steal, both from you and your grandchildren. Just because it hasn't happened yet doesn't mean it won't in the future. Emily and Carter Petersen came home to find their jewelry gone; they had a lock on their bedroom door, but their son and his drug friends had cleaned them out. Nor is it uncommon for parents to take their children's welfare or Social Security checks for themselves or to sell their kids' food stamps for drugs. In fact, I know grandparents who sleep with purses and wallets under their pillows so that their adult children can't find them.

Some of the mothers are prostitutes, and their parents (with grandchild in tow) may encounter them "working" and then have to handle the grandchild's question, "Isn't that my mom?" Some mothers just keep having babies, who are then taken away because of abuse or neglect. It sounds harsh, but the same stories come up again and again and again. "We're not beating up on parents," explains one grandpa. "We're trying to save the next generation."[1]

The fallout is fierce. Both you and your grandchildren can feel like pawns in a game without rules. The children continuously get sideswiped by conflicting emotions, and so do you. They love their parents and fantasize about living with them yet feel deep rejection, abandonment, and anger. You love your child and hope she will get her act together, yet you hate her for what she's doing to you and her kids. You may experience waves of fear for your grandchildren, suffer guilt that you may be at fault, and spin pipe dreams about the day when your adult child can parent again. Meanwhile, you argue with your spouse and still give your wayward adult child every opportunity to clean up her act, worrying all the while that the phone will ring one day and it will be the police.

Some grandparents use up all their money and insurance policies trying to get their children into drug programs. Some pray they'll end up in jail, where they'll at least be safe. Others, less hopeful, take out life insurance policies on their children so that if anything happens, at least they'll have money to bury them.

And then there are the dark wishes and unspeakable thoughts. The thing a parent never expects to feel about a child, namely, that you would all be better off if he or she were dead. "She is thirty-six years old," says a Texas grandmother of her drug-addicted daughter. "I have honestly wished that she would OD and let her son have half a chance at a normal life." It is a horrible thing to think, but when you reach your wit's end—when the grandkids are in mental chaos and your life feels like an armed camp—the dark thoughts do surface. The painful truth is this: As permanent and terrible a loss as death is, it can seem like a lucky break to grandparents who have to watch their adult children destroy themselves and their families moment by painful moment.

■ HOW TO COPE

Most adult children are constantly in and out of your life, causing continual disruption. Only you can break the cycle, but it takes determination, fortitude, and a few guiding principles:

• *Set firm rules and stand by them.* These parents may look like adults, but sometimes you have to treat them like children. You have to set the same kind of rules and limits you set with your grandchild, being firm and consistent. You need consequences that are clearly stated, and you need to stand by them. Don't make threats you can't follow through on, or you'll open yourself to endless manipulation. Perhaps you have told your adult son that his friends are not welcome in your house. You may not be willing to kick him out for inviting them over, but you could take his key away. And if despite your warnings you come home and find four of his friends sitting on the couch, watching television, and drinking beer, you may have to have the locks changed to keep your consequences. But do it. Otherwise, your adult children get the message that even if you talk big, they can still take advantage of you.

• *Learn to say no.* Ruth Castle has a sign on her refrigerator. It says, "NO is a complete sentence." You have to learn to say no to your adult child for the sake of your grandchild. You cannot give your grandchild a stable home if you and your household are at the beck and call of an unstable parent. Your adult child will ask, plead, and demand all kinds of things from you: "Can I borrow the car?" "Can you lend me $20?" "Can you send me supplies in jail?" She will take and take until you have no money left to give, and she will leave you emotionally drained.

Not only is it okay to say no to your adult child, but it is necessary. You will not be abandoning your child; you will be protecting yourself and your grandchildren. Nor do you have to justify yourself. You don't have to give explanations or make speeches. *No* can be a complete sentence.

▪ *Learn to let go.* You need to come to grips with the fact that you cannot really help or change your adult child. This is probably the hardest reality for a parent to face. No matter what this person has done, he is still your child. You gave birth to him and love him, even if you hate what he does. But you have to let go. "My 18-year-old son was getting caught up in drugs. He's left home because he can't do drugs here. He's homeless, but it was his choice," said one grandmother.[2]

BREAKING THE PATTERN OF ENABLING

"One more chance." It's like the magic ring on the merry-go-round. Adult children beg for it: "Give me one more chance, Mom. I'll get it right this time." Grandparents reach out for it: "she's trying so hard now. If I help her, just this once, maybe she'll make it." Like children on a merry-go-round, they go round and round in circles, trying to catch the magic ring, the one that will make everything better. Unfortunately, there are times when helping someone can actually hurt him; when the chances you give your adult child only allow him to continue destructive—and self-destructive—behavior. In the mental health community this kind of help is called "enabling." When you *enable* your adult child, you are doing more than allowing him to continue his behavior, you are actually assisting him.

Grandparents who enable their adult children often only pour good money after bad. They pay for one drug treatment after another, hoping that each new program will be the one that leads to a cure. Unfortunately, true rehabilitation is rare, and the sad reality is that many addicts don't make it. I have set counseling appointments with many adult children as part of their reunification agreements; most don't show up. Some will clean up their acts for a year, even two years, but then they hit a stress they can't handle and they're back to their old ways. It is true that since I see grandparents in crisis, I don't hear many success stories. But when a person abstains from drug use for one or two years and then falls back, at what point do you trust a success story?

"A sure way to cripple a person is to allow her to sponge off you," says one grandparent. "People who are warm, comfortable, and well fed usually have little motivation to change their lifestyles." At one point Pam Marshall decided to keep Linda away from the baby. "I had to choose," she says. "Either Megan or my daughter. My daughter was an adult. The baby wasn't." But it was still difficult for her. Robert finally had to throw Linda out of the house.

No grandparent gets off this merry-go-round until he or she is good and ready. A support group can give you other people's stories to use as a mirror. It can help you find inner strength to say no and mean it. It can prevent you from spinning in circles as much as you would on your own. But only you know when you're truly tired of chasing chances. Even then, there is that extra inning, that last prayer, that last chance before you call it quits.

When grandparents want to let an adult child come home "one last time," I recommend using a written contract. If the contract is violated, the adult child knows that he has to leave.

Try a Written Contract

Verbal promises are tricky; adult children can claim you never told them something or that they didn't understand. Verbal contracts get renegotiated at each stumbling block and have more holes than a colander. With a written contract, everyone knows where they stand. The conditions and consequences are in black and white. By signing the contract all parties are indicating that they understand and agree to accept the consequences if they violate the terms of the contract.

Creating a written contract is like making a behavior chart or a chore chart for your young grandchild. Your rules must be spelled out in detail (for example, "I cannot sleep until 3 P.M.; I must help with the dishes"). It is not enough for a rule to state that the adult child must "find a job in a month." Be specific: "You must not sleep in. You must be out looking for a job from 8:00 A.M to 5:00 P.M., and you must provide me with a list of the employers you have contacted." Otherwise, the adult child could be out all day but spending that time at the movies or in the park.

Each contract item should have its own consequence, one related to the severity of the problem. For instance, if your daughter runs up a $200 phone bill, she can't use the phone until the bill is paid back. I know grandparents who lock the phone in their bedroom so their adult child can't use it. However, your consequences must be realistic. Try not to threaten your adult child with things that you know in your heart you can't do. If the consequence of stealing from you is moving out within 24 hours and if you can't bring yourself to enforce that, then your child will have won. She will immediately start to manipulate you and to ignore her commitments to the contract. The purpose of the contract is to provide incentives to change. If you keep threatening to put your son out but you don't follow through or you let him back two days later, why shouldn't he take $100 from your drawer? Be realistic. What consequences would you really be able to follow through on? Enforcing a contract with your adult child depends entirely on your own ability and willingness to follow through.

Make sure everyone has a copy of the contract. If it is in black and white, no one can misconstrue the rules. Adult children can't say "You never said that" or "I thought you meant such and such." They've read it. They've signed it. There is no gray area. But you must follow through with the consequences or your contract is worth nothing. (See pp. 69–71 for a sample contract.)

Tough Love: One Grandma's Story

"I want my baby to love me. I can't live without my baby," croons Maggie Butler, imitating all the grandparents who can't let go of their adult children. "That's the hook," she says seriously. Maggie knows. She gave her son one last chance to pull himself together, then she finally put him out for good. It was a hard choice. "There is loss there," she admits. "We all lose."

Maggie knew, clearly, that her son's life was in shambles. David was an alcoholic and a drug addict. His marriage had failed years ago, and his two daughters lived in Pittsburgh with his ex-wife and a boyfriend who Maggie suspected was sexually abusing the girls. David had been in and out of detox several times, to no avail, and he had just served two years in jail in West Virginia for assault. But when David's ex-wife abandoned the children on the street one day, he decided to shape up and get custody of his kids. He asked his parents to help him, and they said yes.

Maggie had already done years of work on letting go. She had joined Alanon when she finally accepted the fact that David was an addict; she had gone on to participate in other 12-step programs and had used support groups, as well as individual therapy, in her search to understand herself, her son, and the patterns of addiction. "I had already released David and accepted that he's very much on his own," she said. "But, for some reason, I needed to help him one more time. I said to myself that as his mother I would like to see David get his life together and maybe get his children." It turned out to be a costly lesson: expensive, painful, and emotionally draining.

Since the court would not allow the children to live with David yet, the girls were placed in temporary foster care. David came home, but there were strict terms. He had to go to Alcoholics Anonymous meetings, he had to work, and he could not just sit and watch television. "We will help you," Maggie told him, "but you must help yourself. If you mess up, you're out of here." He said, "Mom, I want to change my life."

When David first came home, he was "good as gold." He got a job at five dollars an hour, although he had once earned three times that amount. He saved his money and bought a car. He got his driver's license, insurance, and a bank account. He made his parole appointments, and he went to meetings religiously for four months. Then something seemed to change. "I think it was just too much good," Maggie says sadly.

One night Maggie's husband went to a meeting David was supposed to attend. He wasn't there. Later, when her son came home, Maggie asked him how the meeting went. "Great," he told her. She didn't say anything, but she was watchful. She was still hoping he would make it. A few days later he went out and didn't come home. He was gone most of the next day, too. That was the last straw for his mother. As she tells it: "He pulls up at six o'clock like a kid with a hand in the cookie jar. 'I guess I messed up, Mom,' he says. 'I guess I should go in and pack.' I said, 'No, your stuff is packed.' That was the deal."

Five days later, after a three-day cocaine binge, David was arrested for kidnapping, robbery, and assault. He was sentenced to 22 years in prison. He was 26.

Maggie now has her granddaughters living with her. She hasn't spoken to David since then, although he writes to her from jail. She loves David, but she chooses not to be in his life right now. She describes herself as a "hard cookie," but it has been a painful process—a lot of grieving, a lot of crying, a lot of letting go. "I used to pray a lot for David," she says. "Now I pray for myself. David will make his own choices. What I have learned from all these support groups is that we have to allow our children to do what they need to do. They have to make all the mistakes. They have to be the ones to pick themselves up. They have to be the ones to find help for themselves. They will always stay crippled if we are the ones to pick them up.

"I have to give up the control and give him the right to live," says Maggie. "Years ago, I said to him, 'David, when are you going to hit your bottom?' He said, 'Mom, I may not have a bottom.'"

Kicking Out Your Adult Child

Putting your child out is the toughest thing in the world. Maggie had 12 years of self-help groups and therapy behind her, and it was still incredibly painful. Some grandparents can't do it until they reach the end of their rope, and even then they need a lot of support. Everyone's bottom line is different. For the Smiths it might be that their son came out of a drug treatment program and relapsed. But the Joneses may still be trying to help a daughter who has been in 16 drug treatment programs and has stolen the car, the jewelry, and the VCR. Each grandparent has a different threshold for feeling that he or she has done everything possible. My rock bottom and your rock bottom can be miles apart.

Some grandparents will talk about the same issues for years and still be unable to act on them. A lot depends on how much support you have from friends and family and how much control you have over your grandchildren. If you kick out the parents, will they—and can they legally—take the child with them? The answer to that question will affect how long it takes you to kick a parent out of the house.

Even after you hit bottom, the obstacles are tremendous. You may find yourself facing guilt, embarrassment, and your own protective feelings. This is, after all, your baby. You gave life to and raised this child, and even if this is not what you brought her up to be, she is still your kid. You might not like this person, but on some level you do love her. Then there are the fears: "Where will my child be? On a park bench? In an alley? Will I get a call to identify a body found in an alley someplace?"

You may also confront strong family pressure: relatives who don't approve of or understand your decision; a spouse who isn't supportive and who undermines your efforts; the grandchildren themselves, who won't understand and who may blame you and cry, "Don't kick out my Mommy! She has no place to go!"

I have seen grandparents who, with support, have managed to let go. Some, like Maggie, pack up their children's belongings and leave them on the porch. Others give their son or daughter a deadline for getting out. Either way, once you tell a child to leave, watch carefully. You might consider changing the locks, in case your child gave copies of the key to friends. Never say, "My child will never do that to me," because you never know. The drugs take control, or friends and lovers exert influence. One couple came home and discovered that their furniture and possessions had been sold. These are things you don't think about until they happen.

Some grandparents persuade their children to move out by setting up apartments for them. They may pay just the first month's rent and deposit, or they may go further and pay the rent and utilities and buy the furniture. It's something many grandparents would like to do, if they could afford it. It is one way for grandparents to get a child out of the house and still reassure themselves that he or she is safe. It's a nice idea; unfortunately, I have rarely seen it work. What I have seen, instead, is this: The apartment gets destroyed; the child invites friends over to "party," sells the furniture for drugs, and eventually gets evicted, often leaving the grandparents with financial liability.

Then there are the adult children who won't leave or who leave but won't stay away. You change the locks and come home to find them on the couch eating ice cream and watching television, the window broken behind them. One grandparent had to go through the eviction process with her own daughter because the police would not evict her.

If you have legal custody of your grandchildren and the parents pose a threat to you or your grandchild, you may be able to get a temporary restraining order against them. How much good it does is debatable. Dorcas King used one to keep her drug-addicted daughter at least 100 feet from her house. Other grandparents have had less success. One thing is certain: It is difficult to call the police on your own child. But if you must, a restraining order may increase your credibility. Remember, you cannot get a restraining order against a parent who has legal custody.

However, all the techniques in the world will be useless until you are ready to let go.

THE CHALLENGE OF CHANGE

Doug and Jane Sullivan's daughter, Mindy, is 28 years old and mentally unstable. She has three children from three different fathers, and her parents are raising them. She started running away at 13 and lived on the street for years. Her parents don't know if she used drugs. Right now she is living at home, but she interferes with the house more than she helps. Once, when Jane asked her to watch the children for an hour, she came back to a house in shambles. Mindy had put the seven-year-old in charge of the little ones and was lying on the couch watching television. The children adore her, but she can't take them for more than two hours.

Mindy repeatedly has horrendous outbursts. She is abusive to everyone in the house. She gets angry at the younger children and swears she will put them in foster care. She tells them they'll never see Grandma and Grandpa again. Once she actually called the police and said, "I want to get rid of my kids." The whole family tiptoes around her. Mindy orders Doug and Jane around like she's the queen of the house and they're her servants. "We spend all our effort and our money and energy on these children, and she doesn't want to help," says Jane. "Unless you watch it, she takes control of the household."

Jane and Doug have made some progress. They now take the kids and leave when Mindy blows up. She still has her outbursts, but at least the children aren't subjected to her threats. This is not the ideal choice. It basically tells Mindy that she can do what she wants and that her parents will leave instead of making her leave. It enables her to continue with the same behavior. However, it does protect the children from her abuse. Until Doug and Jane are ready and able to have their child move out, avoidance is the best choice they have.

Doug and Jane don't lack resolve as much as they are caught in a complex struggle with change. Throughout this chapter we have talked about changing behavior, saying no, setting limits, and even putting your adult child out of the house. But change is never simple. We always have good reasons to change our actions; less apparent are the good reasons not to. To quote psychologist and author Harriet Goldhor Lerner, Ph.D., "Change requires courage, but the failure to change does not signify the lack of it."[3] It took a lot of courage for Maggie to kick her son out of her house. But Jane and Doug, and grandparents like them, don't lack courage. They are still weighing the cost between giving in and giving up. There is a clear benefit to setting limits, but there is also a cost. For most grandparents still struggling with these decisions, the issues at stake are love and fear.

When Love Is at Stake

Love is powerful stuff, and Jane and Doug love Mindy. They raised her, they had hopes for her, and they desperately want to see her get better. Like many grandparents, they are not yet ready to let go. No parent wants to give up the hope that one more chance will save a child. Even 15 or 20 chances later, some grandparents are still trying. A family can deal with these issues for 20 years. When you spend a lifetime loving your child, who can say how many chances it takes to let go of her? There is no magic number. It may take two years in a grandparent support group to get one small change in a grandparent's behavior, but that alone can be a significant thing. Remember, each small change builds a path for bigger change. Until you can make larger strides, keep taking whatever steps you can.

When Fear Is at Stake

Fear is also a powerful motivator, and Doug and Jane are afraid of Mindy. They are afraid she could make good on her threats and disappear with the children. She has done it before. Like many grandparents, Doug and Jane have uncertain custody arrangements. Mindy could easily take her children and wander the streets with them. The grandparents would have nothing to say about it. The only way they can protect their grandchildren is to have them in their home, which means having Mindy there, too. They put up with the mother's behavior for the sake of the children.

Fear and uncertainty are common problems for grandparents who don't have legal custody. They feel trapped and may give in to all kinds of behavior, including extortion or blackmail, to protect their grandchildren. Living without legal custody is like living in an armed camp, always looking over your shoulder; it makes setting limits difficult. If you have this problem, consider what small changes you can make to create pockets of safety for your family. Jane and Doug's leaving with the children when Mindy flies off the handle is their attempt to make the best of a bad situation. Until you are ready or able to make bigger changes, you can only make the best of your situation.

DAMAGE CONTROL: PROTECTING GRANDCHILDREN FROM THEIR PARENTS

As painful as it is for you to witness and suffer the results of your adult child's behavior, it is even harder for your grandchildren. This is, after all, their mother or father, the supposed guardian and architect of their young world. They don't have the age or experience to judge their parent's behavior; they can only react to it and be shaped by it. Chapter 6 will look at the emotional and behavioral problems your grandchildren may face as a result of their circumstances. Here, however, are a few of the questions and problems you may encounter when your adult child interacts with your grandchildren.

What Do I Tell the Kids about Their Parents?

What to tell children and how much to tell them are tough questions for grandparents, and I have heard all kinds of stories about how people have handled this issue. Some grandparents tell the kids that Mom is sick and needs help. Others don't tell them anything, or say they don't know. One grandmother I know tells her grandchildren that Mom and Dad are on vacation whenever the parents land in jail.

I do not advocate lying to children. First of all, they may not believe you. Children pick up on things; they know when secrets are being kept from them. Second, if they do believe you, they will grow up with a distorted view of what life is all about (e.g., that it is common to spend a lot of time on vacation). But, more importantly, if you try to protect children by lying to them and they find out the truth, they'll start to wonder what else you're not telling them.

My parents didn't tell Kevin that my sister committed suicide. They told him she died of a breathing sickness. Later they said she died from smoking too much. Kevin accepted their explanations without question, and as he got older, he assumed his mother had died of lung cancer. When he finally did learn the truth, he was angry. "I felt they lied to me," he said recently. At age 19, the shadow of the lie still lingers. "I don't trust them the same as I might have if they had told me the truth from the beginning. Even if I might not have understood when I was eight, I still would have preferred to know the truth."

Tell the truth, but tell it in bite-size pieces. Think about the child who is asking. How old is he? How much can he understand? What is it that he really wants to know? For example, when a three-year-old asks where babies come from, he's not asking about sex. He just wants to know if he was hatched from a plant or a person. "You came from Mommy's tummy" is all the answer he needs at the moment. This is a conversation a parent will have again and again, over time, as the child's need and ability to understand increase. The same standard applies to grandchildren's questions about their parents. Children need and deserve the truth but in portions they can handle. The answers will depend on their age and maturity, how much contact they have with the parent, what the relationship is with the parent, and what kinds of questions are being asked.

Kids ask a lot of questions that don't require whole explanations: "Where is my mom (or dad)?" "Why can't I be with my parents?" "Will I ever live with my parents again?" Many times grandparents have to admit that they don't know where the parent is. If your grandchild sees her mother, you can tell her Mom has some troubles now. You can reassure her that this is not her fault. If the mother hasn't come by in six years and is remarried in another state, you can tell the child that Mommy is living far away and you don't know when she will come to visit.

Again, consider the age of the child. An eight-year-old will understand that Dad is in jail; a three-year-old doesn't know what jail is. You might tell a very young child that Daddy has gone away and we don't know when he'll be back. As the child gets older, she'll understand more. For instance, Pam Marshall's five-year-old granddaughter, Megan, knows that her mother uses drugs and that drugs make you sick. She knows that Linda's boyfriend hits her, and that's why she isn't allowed to see her mother when he's around. Essentially, she knows enough to understand why she can't do certain things, and in terms that a five-year-old can understand. "We only answer the questions she asks," says her grandmother. "We try to be as honest as we can without burdening too much."

Tell children in pieces, but tell them the truth. They eventually find out, anyway. Children sense a lot of things that they may not be able to verbalize. And be as gentle as possible. These children already have a profound sense of loss, abandonment, and rejection; you don't want to add to that.

What Do I Do When Parents Lie and Make Empty Promises?

Jay and Brenda Saunders are raising their grandson Anthony. Their daughter, Eva, has been abusing cocaine for 25 years. At 40 she is uneducated and homeless; her parents fear she may be selling crack. Eva loves her child dearly, says Brenda, but cannot care for him. "It's a crazy, immature love," she explains. "A child love."

Six-year-old Anthony only lived with his mother for one year, but he adores her. Eva comes to the house and plays with him. She promises to take him away. Sometimes she promises to visit and never shows up; when this happens, she blames other people for the lapse. She also tells her son that Grandma and Grandpa are the reason they can't be together.

Jay and Brenda want Anthony to know his mother. But whenever he sees her, there is a price to pay afterward in regressive behavior or anger at his grandparents. "When she's at the house, we are invisible," Brenda explains. "You can't believe the difference. But when he's with her . . . it's a disaster later on. I think he's furious at both of us because we're not his mother." And it's clear that Anthony suffers. "He's torn," says Brenda. "It's visible. It looks like he's been ripped apart after his mom was here."

Parents promise things: "I'll take you to live with me." "We'll have a house with a dog." "I'll take you bike riding on Sunday." When parents break promises, you get the fallout. Your grandchildren can't help it; you're an easy target. First, because you're there and the parent often isn't. Second, because their feelings about their parents are so conflicted that it is safer to get mad at you.

Broken promises are hard on children, who nevertheless continue to believe in their parents. They wait expectantly for the package or check or for Dad to pick them up at school, and they suffer deeply when nothing happens. Broken promises are equally painful for grandparents, who have to watch their grandchildren suffer each new disappointment as deeply as the first. If you are able to talk to the parents, try to explain the effect of this on the child. Perhaps they can run their plans by you first. If you have legal custody, you can even insist that this happen.

You can also talk to the children. Let them express their feelings about what happens with Mom or Dad. Sometimes they don't want to admit that there's a problem. As they get older, they sometimes come to realize that this is the pattern, that they can't believe what their parents say. Either way, they have strong feelings to express and need safe places to share them. Look to support groups, social workers, and family therapists for feedback about this kind of situation. There is rarely one best way to handle it.

Parents may also lie to their children: "Grandma took you away from me." "Don't listen to Grandpa." "Misbehave with your grandparents, and you can come home." They try to channel their anger and frustration through the children, who don't know whom or what to believe. Lies are even harder for a grandparent to handle. You can't control what a parent tells a child when you're not there, and you don't want to get into debates with your grandchildren about their parents. The best thing you can do is understand the fallout, give the children room to have their reactions, and continue to assure them that they are safe and loved in your home.

Again, if you can prevent the parents from making plans with the child, do; have them make plans with you instead. Tell Mom that you'll be in the park from two to three o'clock, or arrange to meet Dad at the movies. If the parents show up, great. If not, you'll be disappointed, but the child won't be devastated.

What If I Suspect Abuse during Parental Visits?

Continued abuse is a serious concern for many grandparents. Your grandchild may live with you but still have continued contact with unstable or abusive parents. What you can do about it depends on how much control you have over visitation. If you have legal custody of your grandchild and if visitation is at your discretion, you can insist on supervised visits. On the other hand, if court orders call for unsupervised visits and your grandchild comes home with unexplained bruises, contact your social worker immediately. If you suspect any kind of abuse during visits, at least keep a log of what you see and hear, including pictures if you can. Any documentation you gather could be important if a social worker or court becomes involved (see the section "Documentation" later in this chapter for more details).

WHEN THE PARENT IS IN JAIL

Handling your adult child is somewhat easier when she is in jail. As painful as it is, you know your child is safe and you know that, for the moment, she cannot physically disrupt your life or that of your grandchild. But the fact that your child is out of sight does not put her out of mind or out of contact with you. You may get frequent collect calls and letters requesting money for cigarettes and shampoo. Even at a distance, your child can play on your heartstrings. Be careful. If your child says she needs something and you do want to help out, send the item, not the money. Here, too, think about whether you are really helping or only enabling.

The picture changes when the adult child is about to be released from jail. Some will ask to come home at that time. If yours does, and you want her to come home, do not send money; send a nonrefundable ticket instead. I have seen several situations in which grandparents sent money for a bus or a train ticket for an adult child to come home. They prepared the grandchild to see the mother or father, and the parent never came. Instead, he or she hooked up with old friends and cashed the ticket in. The child and the grandparents were devastated.

This is exactly what happened to Marta Sobol, a grandmother from Poland. Her oldest daughter, Anna, had been in and out of jail and rehab while Marta raised Anna's eight-year-old son, Christopher. Anna was now in jail again and started to write her mother lengthy letters of remorse. She had changed, she said. She wanted to be a good mother; she wanted to know her child, to be a real parent to him; and she wanted another chance. Marta didn't want to give in, but Christopher, always hopeful, begged his grandmother to give his mother another chance. I talked with Marta for months in GAP meetings, preparing her for the possibility that Anna might be using her again and making empty promises to Christopher. Finally, the time arrived. Marta sent Anna a bus ticket and told her that she and Christopher would be at the station. As soon as she saw her, Marta knew her daughter wasn't serious. After all her repentant letters, Anna had made arrangements to have friends pick her up. "I'm going out for a little while," she told her son. "I'll see you when I get home tonight." The child fell asleep at 10:00 P.M. and woke up again at 2:00 A.M., sobbing because Mom wasn't back yet. She never came back. She ended up back in jail after seeing her son for 10 minutes at the bus station.

Barbara Douglas had a similar story. Her daughter, Rhonda, had supposedly recovered in jail and wanted a fresh start. Barbara and her husband, offering to give her one more chance to come home, sent a ticket. The day she was released, Rhonda called to say she would be home the next morning, after she went to get her belongings. Barbara said, "Don't go anyplace. Don't pick up anything. We'll buy you new clothes, whatever you need. We'll start you over. Just come home." She didn't want Rhonda to go back to her old place because she knew that Rhonda's friends would get to her and that she wouldn't be strong enough to say, "No, I don't do this anymore." Rhonda didn't listen, and Barbara only heard from her months later, when she was once again in jail. At that point Barbara and her husband filed for guardianship of their grandson.

Some adult children don't even make a pretense of coming home; they go directly to their old neighborhoods and friends. Their parents may not hear from them again until they're back in jail. One day they get another collect call, and the cycle starts again.

Nevertheless, there are those who truly recover in prison. They get involved in Alcoholics Anonymous or some other program and start to put their lives together. But successful rehabilitation depends on how long an individual is incarcerated and how willing he is to change. Unfortunately, I have seen few cases of successful recovery. More often, I see adult children make empty promises and revert to old habits.

Remember, if there is no court order giving you legal custody of your grandchild, either through dependency or guardianship proceedings, a parent may resume custody when he or she is released from prison. If you have concerns about your grandchild and the system is not involved, you might consider seeking guardianship while the parent is incarcerated (see Chapter 10).

WHEN A DAUGHTER KEEPS HAVING BABIES

Julia Stone's daughter has already lost custody of four children; now she is pregnant again. "We all think maybe it will go away," Julia says quietly. It's a terrible thing to be a mother with a pregnant daughter and to be praying for a miscarriage. But that seems to be the only thing to do when your daughter keeps having babies—often drug babies—she can't care for. You can't force her to use birth control, and you certainly can't reason with her. Yet there are grandparents who are raising as many as six or seven children from the same mother. The babies are all medically fragile, and they just seem to keep coming—partly because the mothers know Grandma will care for them and partly because the mothers don't think about it at all.

The young women who have baby after baby aren't thinking about repercussions or about the fact that they already have five drug-addicted children out there. They are thinking about immediate gratification: the next man, the next fix. Often they are prostituting themselves without precautions. They could get an IUD or contraceptive implant, but they aren't able to plan ahead or follow through. Marlena Hunt's daughter scheduled an appointment for a tubal ligation but was back in jail before she could make the visit. Sandra Cobb's daughter planned to have her tubes tied after her sixth pregnancy but she delivered in a Catholic hospital and they wouldn't perform the surgery. Before she could get around to it, she was pregnant again.

Even the ones who may not be on drugs but who may be mentally unstable are not thinking about birth control. Liz Andersson's family has a history of mental illness, and her daughter inherited the problem. She is not responsible enough to take birth control measures, won't do a tubal ligation, and has already had five sons, ranging in age from 12 years to 18 months. Liz, who is 65, is raising them all.

Some women seem to have children just for the welfare check. I know there are many parents with large families who live just below the poverty level; that doesn't mean they are using drugs or neglecting their children. The parents I'm referring to are the ones who keep having kids but don't parent them. Often there are drugs involved. These are the mothers whose parents are already raising two or three of their children. If the grandparents get government aid for the children, the daughter may have her "own" baby to get welfare. Women who prostitute themselves for drug money may also get pregnant. If the choice is between paying for an abortion or getting welfare benefits during and after the pregnancy, they may have (and keep) the baby—until this one, too, gets removed by the courts. In the mind of a drug-addicted mother, a baby may mean easy cash for drugs.

Some mothers are even self-righteous about their children. One young woman I heard about had seven children taken away from her by the system before she was 30. The last one was removed when she threatened to push him in front of a truck—and she is sure the system is at fault!

Unfortunately, there isn't much you can do when a daughter keeps having babies. The options aren't encouraging. You can keep taking them, although your finances and energy may already be stressed to the limit. You can try to encourage her to get her tubes tied or get a contraceptive implant, but it must be her choice. Or you can let the next one go into foster care. Wanda Davis is one grandmother who managed to make that decision. She only has one of her four grandchildren, her sister is raising one, and two more are in the foster care system. Diane Snyder also has one grandchild, her sister has another, one was put up for adoption, and Mom has the fourth. Still, as much as you tell yourself you won't take the next one, when that baby comes, it's hard. Sandra Cobb has said that many times; she is now 67 years old and is raising seven grandchildren from the same daughter, ranging in age from 2 to 14 years.

One thing you can do is realize that you have no control over your daughter and make peace with what you will or will not do when the next baby arrives. Be realistic about your circumstances and your ability to say no. Your decision is not just about what is best for that baby but what is best for the children you already have and what is best for you. Remember, if you don't protect yourself, you can't protect even one grandchild. Consider what decisions you can live with and make peace with them.

When Mom Has Another Child and Keeps It

There are a number of reactions your grandchildren could have if their mother keeps the next baby; these depend on their age and the degree of contact they have with her. Two common reactions, however, are abandonment and relief.

A child who wants to be with his mother can be totally devastated if Mom has another baby. Feelings of low self-esteem and abandonment are compounded, and the child may wonder, "Why is she having another baby if I'm already here? If she can take care of a baby, why isn't she taking care of me?" He may lash out in anger and may regress to bed-wetting, thumb-sucking, and using baby talk in an effort to become a baby again so Mom will take care of him.

On the other hand, a child who is secure with Grandma and Grandpa might be relieved that Mom has another baby. She may think, "Maybe now Mom will leave me alone." The child may, in fact, feel guilt or anxiety about being safe with you while the new baby is with her mother. A child who is well settled with you might be afraid of being taken away. Unfortunately, you can never guarantee children that they will never be removed, unless you have adopted them. Even legal guardianship can be revoked.

DOCUMENTATION

Emily Petersen saved everything connected with her granddaughter—pictures, letters, birthday cards—because she thought she might need them someday. Lucy Davis kept a notebook documenting every visit with her daughter-in-law, whether it was good, bad, or even a no-show. She wrote down everything that happened and her granddaughter's reactions to each event. She knew that her memory alone would not be enough if she wanted to recount these things later on. Each of these grandmothers came to bless her foresight.

When Emily's granddaughter Amanda was three years old, the child's mother (Emily's daughter-in-law) asked Emily and Carter to adopt her. Sheila became less cooperative, however, as the adoption proceeded, and told the social worker handling the case that neither she nor her parents were ever allowed to see Amanda. It wasn't true, and Emily could prove it. She had cards and letters from Sheila thanking her for watching Amanda and for letting her see her child, as well as photos of the other grandparents at the house for Easter. Her careful documentation put Sheila's accusations in perspective.

Lucy, on the other hand, found herself facing an angry judge. Lucy had canceled visitation one afternoon because Lindsey started vomiting when she heard she had to see her mother. "Who do you think you are?" demanded the judge, who assumed she was arbitrarily refusing parental visits. "Here," Lucy said, pulling out her notebooks. "It is all here. She had thirty-two scheduled visits; she showed up for twelve." The judge agreed that visitation had to be consistent or not at all and ordered that future visits be held at the courthouse in order to monitor the mother's attendance.

Even if you're not currently involved with the system, document everything. If at some point in the future you do find yourself involved with the court or even a private attorney, you may have less of an ordeal if you have records of the parents' behavior and the children's reactions to parental visits. You look more organized and accurate if you have information written down in concrete detail and chronological order. If you have to rely on your memory, your statement to the judge may go something like this: "My daughter drops by unexpectedly and intoxicated. The last visit was maybe six or ten weeks ago." Compare that statement with: "On June 14 my daughter appeared at my door unannounced. She was staggering and slurring her speech." It makes a much better impression in court, and you don't have to rely on your own memory.

How to Document

- Keep a journal or log. Use a bound diary or calendar, and keep a daily record of your adult child's behavior and anything pertaining to your grandchildren. Don't use a loose-leaf notebook; a bound book is a much more convincing document because the chronological order cannot be faked.
- Don't write down what you *think* is happening, only what you can verify with dates, times, and photos. It is one thing to say, "My daughter never visits when she promises to." It is another to say, "On May sixth my daughter said she would come for a visit on May seventh; that was six weeks ago, and we haven't heard from her since."—especially when you have the calendar entries to prove it.
- Write down everything concerning the parent: the time, day, and nature of phone calls and visits; the child's behavior and reactions before, during, and after the call or visit; and the behavior of the parent. Does the parent appear to be in control or under the influence of something when he calls or comes

by? Does the parent ask about the child when he calls? How often does the parent call? Does he visit as promised? Does the parent make promises that aren't kept—ice cream, toys, birthday presents, trips? Write it all down.

- Document what the parent *doesn't* do: when she doesn't visit, doesn't show, doesn't call, doesn't send a card for a birthday or holiday.
- Record everything you spend on the child and keep receipts. This not only verifies what it costs you to keep the child, but could be used later to prove that Mom and Dad are not supporting him.
- Document everything that might be helpful to show a court that the parent is not ready to handle the responsibility of raising a child. If a child comes back from a visit with a parent and has unexplained bruises or resumes bed-wetting or thumb-sucking after being with Mom or Dad, write it down. Write everything down.
- Be forewarned: having documentation won't guarantee a positive court response. I know grandparents who had everything written down but were not permitted to enter their journals as evidence, and I know grandparents whose records, though presented to the court, didn't help. Still, it is better to have records and not be able to use them than to need records and not have them. And if you do get the opportunity to present information, you will look more organized and believable if everything is documented.

Sample Written Contract

The Story

Donna and Hal Smith are raising two grandsons. Their daughter Caroline is 31 years old, divorced, and drug addicted. She has been through numerous drug treatment programs, and she has been in jail several times. Each time she is released, she makes and then breaks the same promises. She has stolen her mother's jewelry and even her kids' piggy bank to buy more drugs. Now she is coming out of rehab again, and her parents want to give her one last chance for the sake of the children. This time,

(continued)

(continued from previous page)

however, they are using a written contract, signed by Caroline and witnessed by their family therapist.

The Contract

Rules of the House

Between Donna and Hal Smith and Caroline Black.

The purpose of this contract is so that we can all live peacefully under the same roof and know what our expectations are of each other.

For Caroline Black to continue to live with Donna and Hal Smith, the following rules must apply. These are not in order of importance.

1. Caroline must strive to lead a sober and productive life. She must prove to her parents that she can be a good mother and a safe provider for her children. She is not to socialize with any of her old friends from the street.

2. This phone number is only to be given out on job applications. Donna or Hal will take all calls. Caroline may use the phone only with permission from Donna or Hal, or she will lose her phone privileges.

3. Caroline must be in this residence by 10:30 P.M. or call by 10:00 if she can't make it on time. She is not to be in the house alone, unless given permission by Donna or Hal. Caroline is not allowed to take any property from this residence unless given permission by Donna or Hal. Caroline shall not give out this address to anyone (unless it pertains to a job). The doors of the house and garage are to be kept locked at all times. Electricity and water are to be used only as needed.

4. Caroline is to start an outpatient drug program immediately. She is expected to comply with any drug testing required by her parole officer or by Donna or Hal. Caroline must also start a counseling program to help begin a new relationship with her children. These counseling sessions must be attended weekly. Alcoholics Anonymous or Narcotics Anonymous programs must be attended three times a week.

5. Caroline is expected to find a job within two months. She may not sleep in. She must be out looking for a job from

(continued)

(continued from previous page)

8:00 A.M. to 5:00 P.M. and must provide her parents with a list of employers she has contacted. Once she has a job, she must then contribute to the expenses of running the house. This includes food and monthly bills.

6. Donna and Hal are to provide food and shelter to Caroline. They will give Caroline a bus pass, but they will not give Caroline any money. Donna and Hal are not responsible for Caroline's transportation.

7. Caroline must share in household responsibilities. She must cook dinner three times a week and do dishes on the other nights. She must do her children's laundry, pack their school lunches, and keep her own room clean.

8. Caroline must not upset her children. She must realize that her children come first, and she may not raise her voice or spank them. She is not to make promises to her children or plans without discussing them with Donna or Hal first. She may not take the children away from the house without supervision.

9. At any time, Donna and Hal have the right to ask Caroline to leave if they think she is under the influence of any drug or alcohol.

10. Caroline must leave this residence if any of these rules are broken. Caroline must also leave if she cannot live by the rules of this contract. This is a firm contract between Donna and Hal Smith and Caroline Black. The purpose of this contract is to restore Donna and Hall's trust in Caroline Black and to assure the safety of Caroline's children.

11. At the advice of Donna's counselor, Martha Steven, Donna and Hal must keep this contract in force.

(Date) _____ Caroline Black

_____ Donna Smith

_____ Hal Smith

witnessed by _____ Martha Steven

A reminder: This is only a sample contract. Your own contract should reflect your own needs and purpose. However, try to write it with tight rules and specific expectations. Then, as trust is restored, you can loosen up a little. It is much more difficult to start loose and then have to tighten the rules later on.

CHAPTER 6

Your Troubled Grandchild

> You raise your kids; you think it's over. No one
> tells us it's just the beginning.
>   —*Colorado grandmother*

One morning when John and Carol Waters's daughter didn't answer the phone, John crawled in her window and found her dead in her bed with her three-year-old son in her arms. The little boy was desperately trying to wake his mother, who had died of a heart attack in her sleep. When I first met this family, Brian was so insecure he could not let Grandma sit in a chair beside him; he had to sit in her lap and would have crawled inside her if he could have. Grandma couldn't be out of his sight even to go to the bathroom. She had to sleep in his room. Brian couldn't sleep through the night and was constantly telling Grandma not to close her eyes. He was afraid that if she fell asleep, she, like his mother, would never wake up.

Carolyn Parker's grandson, Eric, had been living on the streets with his drug-addicted teenage mother. One day the young woman left the little boy alone in a motel room, and neighbors called child protective services, who called Carolyn. He was like "a wild animal" when he arrived, says Carolyn. At two years the child could barely talk; he only cried and screamed. He didn't know how to sit down and eat properly, and he was painfully insecure; he hoarded food and screamed every time anyone tried to take his new coat away. "He thought he wouldn't get it back," says Carolyn. "He had nothing he could call his."

Four-year-old Heather Pierce was a very sad, frightened little girl when she arrived at her grandmother's house. She wet her bed, she hid under the cushions on the couch, and she had trouble sleeping. But she wasn't afraid of the dark. Instead, she was afraid of the light. She needed everything shut and tightly closed—the windows, the blinds, the door—and complete darkness before she could fall asleep at night. She was afraid that her father, who was in prison for murdering her mother, would come and get her, too.

Not only are you raising a child you never planned for, but you may be raising a child with multiple problems. Many of these children are the walking wounded. They are good kids, but they have not had a good start in life. They may be anxious and insecure. Since the people who were supposed to nurture them have, through choice or accident, left them, they may have a tough time trusting anyone or anything. Many have been left alone in motels and in strangers' homes. They may be used to falling asleep in one place and waking up somewhere else. They have no sense of stability.

Some of the children will defy authority. Some have been responsible for themselves since they were five or six years old. They may have cared for infant siblings, diapering and feeding them; they may have cared for drug-addicted parents. They think they can come and go as they please. Far from grateful, these kids may resent your taking on the role of parent and may rebel when you set rules.

Some grandchildren are physically and verbally aggressive— with you, other adults, and other children. They only know how to get negative attention and may fight, swear, lie, and even commit petty crimes to get noticed. They will push your limits to see how far they can go until you finally push them away. Since everyone else has abandoned them, they reason, it's only a matter of time before you do, too. Children who have been molested may act out sexually, and even very young children will pick up inappropriate sexual behavior if they have been exposed to pornography or have seen their mothers with various men.

On the other hand, your grandchildren might be the best-behaved youngsters, sturdy little ones who seem to have it all together. You may even count on them to help you with their younger siblings. But an excesssivly mature and obedient child is also a source of worry. For healthy, normal development children need their childhood, and that means acting like children. Some of these children may also withdraw and get depressed. They turn their feelings inward and become introspective and shy, isolating themselves from adults and peers. They're your "easy" kids. But don't let this behavior fool you; they may be just as needy as children who overtly act out.

The tricky thing in all of this is that three children who have had the same neglectful upbringing or the same traumatic loss could react in three completely different ways.

WHAT YOUR GRANDCHILD IS FEELING

To understand your grandchild's behavior, it helps to understand what he or she is going through. In the turmoil of a shattered family, children are the most affected and the least prepared to understand or talk about it. A small child can't turn around and say, "I am angry because my mother abandoned me, and I'm afraid it might be my fault." Instead, she may act out her feelings. She may become aggressive at school or depressed and withdrawn; she may have difficulty sleeping, wet her bed, or revert to baby talk. The types of emotional problems a child experiences and their severity will depend on the individual child, on how much trauma she survived, and on the child's age and stage of development when she moves in with you. However, most grandchildren will experience a similar set of intense, overlapping feelings.

Grief and Abandonment

Every case of grandparents raising grandchildren is somehow about loss—for the grandparent and the grandchild. And where there is loss, grief inevitably follows. Whether a parent is absent owing to death or drugs, these children suffer a profound sense of loss, abandonment, and rejection.

Don't let appearances fool you. Children grieve differently than adults do. They grieve like children. One little boy was four the year his father left and his mother died. When his grandmother took him in, he was "a little wildcat." "He suffered a tremendous amount of losses," she says. "Grief in a child is anger."[1]

Nightmares, confusion, and even moments of forgetfulness and joy are also part of a child's grieving process. When my sister died, my mother felt that Kevin wasn't grieving the way he should. He wanted to play with his friends, have a good time. He was trying to put his life back together.

Young children don't have the concept that death is really final. They go from periods of sadness and depression to moments when they block things out. They may not remember what has happened. They may focus on things like toys and friends. They may repeatedly ask if or when Mommy is coming back. The biggest difference between the child who has been orphaned and the one who has been abandoned is the answer to that question. For one, it is certain Mommy is not coming back. Understand, however, that it is normal for children to alternate between overt sorrow and happy self-involvement. It may be hard on you to hear your grandchild's laughter if your own child has just died, but your grandchild is processing the death in his own way. Just as you must mourn at your own pace, allow your grandchild to set the pace for his own grieving process.

There are many books that help children deal with death and that are written on a level they can understand. We used several with Kevin when my sister died, and I highly recommend checking some out at the library (see Appendix A for suggestions).

A child who is orphaned loses his parent once, and it is permanent and tragic. A child whose parents are in jail, in rehab, on the street, or just missing harbors a hope of returning to them but in the meantime loses them over and over again as they wander in and out of the child's life. Strange as it may seem, a sudden death may be easier for a child to handle than months or even years of not knowing. It is the difference between a clean break and prolonged uncertainty, and certainty is extremely important to children.

Reassurance, nurturing, and acceptance are what your grandchild needs, as well as consistency and routine. Children need to be reassured that you will not leave them and that they are safe. These children have a low sense of self-esteem and a high sense of self-blame. Do things to shore up your grandchild's self-image; use positive reinforcement and praise. Remind him over and over that you love and accept him. Predictability and sameness are also important. Try to maintain a consistent, predictable routine so that your grandchild can begin to trust you and his new environment. It takes a while, but it eventually sinks in.

Guilt

Children feel incredible guilt when a crisis happens in the family and a parent is suddenly absent. The crisis can be a divorce, an arrest, a suicide—it doesn't matter. Children have a narrow definition of cause and effect. It is easy for them to believe that the parent would not have left if only they had been "good," if only they had been more helpful, if only they had cleaned their room or finished their dinner. In some distorted way, they blame themselves for their parents' not taking care of them.

The guilt intensifies if a child comes to you from an abusive or neglectful situation. She may feel relieved about being with you and away from her parents, but that same relief feels like a betrayal of her parents. And if she has been placed with you over the wishes of her parents, she may feel like a pawn, split down the middle in her loyalties, caught between her love for her parents and her need to be safe with you. Your grandchild may also feel guilty for being a burden in your life, particularly if she is the cause of friction between you and your spouse. Even when there is no friction, a child may feel guilty for changing your life. "Poor Grandma," six-year-old Lindsey told her aunt. "Daddy is always going to parties. Aunt Dawn and Jason are married now, and they go everywhere. And poor Grandma. . . . You know, she's got me, and she never goes anywhere." "It isn't that I say it," says her grandmother, "but the child is not blind."

It is critical that you help your grandchildren understand that they are not to blame for their parents' absence or the current situation. Again, the key is reassurance and positive reinforcement. You cannot use logic to change children's minds; you can only continually reassure them. Give them affection and frequent praise. One grandmother always looks for something positive to focus on with her hyperactive grandson. Even when he is acting out or misbehaving, she will ask him to take something to the trash for her or to turn on the light; this way she can praise him and continue building his self-esteem.

Anger

Seven-year-old Gabriel is a good kid, but one morning he started throwing things and came after his grandfather with a pipe, saying, "I'm going to kill Grandpa." Yet at the end of the day, he was hugging Grandpa good night. Adam, 15, told his grandmother he would break a window, and he did; he threw his skateboard through it. And four-year-old Monica has started choking cats.

Anger builds up inside children—anger at their parents for not being there or for breaking promises, anger at you for not being their parents, anger at the neglect and abuse they experienced before coming to live with you. They may blame you for sending their parents away (their parents may even tell them that you did). If they had the run of the streets before coming to you, they may also resist your attempts to impose rules, limits, and structure. Very young children lack words and will physically express their feelings, but even older children may act out complex emotions. Grandparents often become the target of the unexpressed anger these children feel, perhaps because the parents are absent or because the children think that if they do express their feelings, their parents will abandon them forever. You're an easy target. Try not to take this personally, however; you are also their lifeline.

Try to direct and channel your grandchild's anger when he gets mad. Help him verbalize his feelings. It is better for a child to say, "I'm mad because my Mommy didn't come to see me today and she promised," than for him to hit someone. Let your grandchild know that it is okay to be angry, that you understand that he feels hurt and confused, but that it is not okay to hit or threaten. Teach the child that feelings and actions are different. If he can't verbalize his feelings, let him get the anger out safely on a pillow or punching bag.

An angry child who threatens someone, even if it is with a plastic baseball bat, has reached a crisis point. It doesn't matter whether or not the threat would have been carried out. The fact that the child was that angry and couldn't channel that feeling is a warning sign. Children who have reached this point could hurt someone; they could also hurt themselves. If the problem isn't addressed, it may only worsen as they get older. Anger that is extreme or disrupts your daily life is a sign of crisis. This is the time to seek professional counseling for the child—and for yourself, so that you can learn to help her.

Fear, Anxiety, and Insecurity

Every child has fears of some sort—of the dark, the boogeyman, being lost. The world is a big place full of dangerous unknowns, and children are particularly powerless in it. But while a night-light can take care of a childish fear of the dark and you can talk about the questionable existence of the boogeyman, what can you do about a child who has already lived the nightmare? Your grandchild knows there are real things to fear because she has seen them. The child may not trust adults because her parents proved untrustworthy. She is probably terrified of being abandoned again, this time by you. "Who will take care of me if Grandma gets sick?" is a scary thought for a kid.

When Marilyn McIntosh first got her grandchildren, they were anxious and insecure. They asked questions like these: "Do you love us as much as you loved your own kids?" "Are you and Grandpa always going to live together?" "Are you going to live long enough for me to grow up and take care of myself?"[2] As time passes and children are exposed to the constancy of a loving, safe environment and a normal, predictable daily routine—having their clothes and toys in the same place each day and sleeping in the same bed every night—the questions come less frequently. But they are probably never far from the surface: Anne Sutter was just flopped across her bed one day, tired after a grueling day at work. Perhaps she dozed awhile. It was enough to panic her six-year-old grandson. Anne woke to a child frantically shaking her foot and yelling, "Mommy! I thought you were dead!"

There are also fears about the parents: "Won't they ever come back?" Or the reverse: "What if they *do* come back?" One little boy was so afraid that his mother would come and take him that he built traps for her; he rigged a gate with rubber snakes so that if she tried to open the gate, the snakes would pop up and scare her away.[3]

Reassuring frightened children takes time, patience, and consistency—not just the consistency of reassuring words and hugs but of three meals a day, regular school hours, a stable routine. You may have to reassure your grandchildren again and again as they slowly adjust to their new situation. Extreme fears, however, may indicate a need for counseling.

Embarrassment

Some children may be sensitive about the fact that they live with grandparents, particularly when other children are around. They may also be embarrassed by their parents. It is difficult for children to accept the fact that their situation is different from that of their peers. Their friends may ask painful questions and tease them. The parents of their friends are probably younger and able to participate in more activities. Although there are increasing numbers of older first-time parents, as well as young grandparents, the age factor can spark embarrassing, if innocent, questions. "Where's your mother?" a little girl in the playground asked seven-year-old Melissa one day. The little girl had heard Melissa call her 70-year-old grandmother "Mommy" and didn't believe mothers had so much gray hair. "Where's your mother?" the little girl persisted. Melissa didn't know how or what to answer. She doesn't know where her mother is—her mother abandoned her when she was 10 months old and she has never seen her. Grandma overheard the exchange and came to her rescue. "Why do you ask so many questions?" she asked the little girl; then she changed the subject.

Perhaps you live in a small community and your grandchild's friends know that the child's parent is in jail or on drugs. The teasing may be far less innocent. Children can be cruel, and they will use whatever ammunition they can find to inflict pain. Fifteen-year-old Vanessa constantly gets into fights at school. The other children say horrible things to her: that her mother was a "jailbird," that her mother didn't want her, that her mother had syphilis. Vanessa says that she gets into fist fights because the taunts make her "crazy."

Sometimes the parent's presence itself is the problem. Sixteen-year-old Mark remembers coming home from shopping one day to find his mother stretched out on the front lawn looking "like a bum." He recalls, "I felt so embarrassed; I never wanted to come back. My friends were standing around and said, 'Who's that?' I said 'Just a friend of the family.' I can't believe I said that. And then someone said, 'That's his mother.' Everybody knew about my mother by then, but nobody ever saw her. And she was lying on the grass, and the neighbors were staring."

These are hard situations to face, and there is no perfect way to handle them. Teach your grandchildren that they don't have to answer questions that make them uncomfortable, that they can change the subject or say, "I don't want to talk about that right now." Teach them to use their words, not their fists, when they are angry. But, most importantly, try not to be hurt by their hurt and embarrassment. When they talk about these feelings at home, it is important to listen and acknowledge their pain. Growing up is hard enough without all these extra problems. What they most need is for you to understand that. You can't make it go away and you can't make it better, but you can certainly hear them.

Hope and Fantasy

Unless they are terrified of them your grandchildren will probably never give up the hope, the fantasy, that their parents will some-day come back and take care of them. Although they love you, the parent–child bond is a tight one that never vanishes–even when a child has been mistreated. Ten-year-old Stephanie was abandoned by her mother when she was two years old. She hasn't seen her in five years, but she still fantasizes about her. One day Stephanie called 911 and asked the sheriff to find her mother. Although five-year-old Marcy was physically and sexually abused, she still talks about going back and living with Mom. Many children want to remain with their grandparents, but they fantasize about having their parents join them. When five-year-old Megan's mother asked Megan if she wanted to live with her, the child replied, "No, I want you to come live with all of us in the same house."

These hopes and fantasies can result in erratic behavior on the part of the child. Some children act out in the hope that their grandparents will be unable to handle them and will send them back to their parents. Others will become depressed and withdrawn. Says one grandmother, "The kids believe their mom will come get them. When it doesn't happen, we get anger." The reverse is also true: Children who are returned to their parents and are unhappy may misbehave so they will be sent back to Grandma's.

It is normal for your grandchildren to have these hopes and dreams and to be disappointed when they don't come true. All you can do is let them know you understand their feelings and that you will continue to be there for them when they need you.

COMMON BEHAVIOR PROBLEMS

Every child who lives with grandparents suffers some part of this emotional kaleidoscope. Children need reassurance that their thoughts and feelings are normal and that most other children in their situation would have similar ones. Encourage your grandchildren to express their feelings in whatever way they can, provided they don't hurt themselves or others in the process. If they can talk about being hurt or angry or frightened, they are less likely to channel those feelings into inappropriate or negative behavior.

Not every child, however, is capable of verbalizing feelings. Sometimes the feelings are too big; sometimes there are too many of them. And many children are too young to understand what they are going through, let alone talk about it.

What follows are some common behavior problems and parenting issues that trouble grandparents. Remember, children act out what they cannot verbalize. These behavior problems are mostly symptoms of underlying emotional issues. Sometimes several behaviors may be related to one issue. For instance, a child who is experiencing eating and sleeping disorders as well as severe "clinginess" may be suffering from a shattered sense of trust and will need your help to restore it. On the other hand, these three behaviors could have three different emotional roots. In any case, both your grandchild's behavior and the feelings behind them will need to be addressed for the child to make a healthy adjustment to his or her new living situation.

Excessive Clinging

Fear and insecurity can make a grandchild excessively clingy. Carol Waters couldn't take a shower without her grandson Brian in the bathroom. He wanted to sit in her lap in public, not next to her. He didn't want to be left at school or with a baby-sitter and cried excessively when she left.

When their grandparents are attending a GAP session, the children will often wander past the door and peek in just to make sure that Grandma or Grandpa is still in the same place. Five-year-old Megan often sleeps in Grandma's lap through the whole session to avoid having to leave her grandmother and go with the other kids. And one day when six-year-old Gregory saw the group members leave the room and his grandmother was not among them—she was in the bathroom—he let out a bloodcurdling scream: "Where is my grandma!?"

Most children have clingy moments, but for these children clinging is almost a way of life. They may also talk excessively as a way of keeping adults not only physically present but also mentally and emotionally present. For a harried grandparent, behavior like this can be hard to handle. Try to understand that your grandchild doesn't want to drive you crazy but is only trying to stay safe. These children are terrified of being left or forgotten, even for a moment. It takes time, reassurance, and consistency for grandchildren to trust again and feel secure. Once they start trusting that you will continue to be there for them, and can see it with their own eyes, the clingy behavior will ease up (although it may reappear again in times of change).

For severe situations like Brian's, however, therapy may be needed. I worked with Carol Waters's grandson Brian in individual and family therapy for several years. At first I had Grandma stay in the office with us for the entire time. Then I told her to say in the middle of the therapy session that she had to go to the bathroom. Brian would scream and yell in a fit of anger and panic. I would hold him at the door of the bathroom while Carol talked to him from the other side. Then she would be silent for a minute and come out. Brian thought she was going to disappear through some secret door in there. He finally reached the point where he could see me without having Grandma in the room and could go off to play in the park with other children during GAP events. But it took time, patience, and a great deal of consistency and reassurance.

Sleeping Problems

Five-year-old Patrick was raised by a mentally ill mother and an abusive father and stepmother before coming to live with his grandmother. He is so frightened and insecure that he can't sleep in his own room; he sleeps on a mat on the floor by Grandma. The same thing happened with Kevin after my sister died. I had temporarily moved in with my parents after graduate school and slept on a mat on the floor next to Kevin's bed. My nephew wouldn't sleep unless I was holding his hand. If I moved at all, he would wake up instantly. If I wasn't there, he would take his blanket in the middle of the night and lie down beside my parents' bed. He was very afraid that people were going to die on him again, and we were all he had.

Sleeping problems are common with children whose lives have been disrupted. They take the form of nightmares, fear of the dark, and wanting to sleep with the grandparents. These are unspoken cries of insecurity and indicate a need for reassurance, nurturing, and trust.

Going to bed can be a difficult time for your grandchild. It means a long separation from you and may tap fears that you could disappear in the night or that she may wake up in a strange environment. Again, reassurance, consistency, and a predictable routine are key. Try to establish a bedtime ritual. Set a bedtime hour and stick to it. As you tuck your grandchild in, talk about how the day went and any plans you may have for tomorrow, letting her know you will be there if she gets scared at night and when she wakes up in the morning. You can even leave a picture of yourself or the family by the bed to reassure her. Bedtime rituals can be a wonderful, secure part of childhood, a time that your grandchild may use to discuss the day or confide in you.

If, on the other hand, you have a grandchild who can't sleep or wakes up with nightmares, there are a number of things you can try to get him back to bed: You can rub his back, sing to him or read him bedtime stories to quiet him down (although you don't want to reward waking up if it becomes a nightly habit). A night-light in the room and hallway can help youngsters who have nightmares. Try to address the problem in the child's room. Children need to feel secure in their own beds, and sleeping alone is an important step in learning a healthy autonomy. Besides, you need your privacy, too. Once you consistently allow a child to sleep in your bed, the habit is more difficult to break.

As children begin to work through their fears and rebuild trust, their sleeping problems should start to dissipate. My nephew Kevin eventually learned to sleep alone in his room, and Heather Pierce has begun to sleep with her windows open. But it takes time, patience, and, with some children, counseling to help them process the trauma and loss they have experienced.

Eating Problems

Food can be the focus of several kinds of problems for your grandchildren. They may not have had enough to eat before they came to you. They may eat too fast or too much, as if each meal might be their last for some time. They may even start hoarding food. When two-year-old Eric arrived at his grandparents' house, he ate so quickly he was in danger of choking. "Eric, take little bites; there's plenty of food," his grandmother would assure him. And six-year-old Daryl hides food under his bed, even cans he can't open.

On the other hand, some children may get depressed and stop eating or may refuse to eat, using mealtime as a way to get your attention. Charlotte Buckley has a four-year-old grandson who turns food into a power struggle. Joey won't take a bite unless Grandma is there to bribe and spoon-feed him; sometimes even that doesn't do any good. He does eventually eat, however, when she ignores him.

When you are dealing with a problem concerning food, whether a child is eating too much or too little, you need to rule out any medical problems. Most likely the problem is related to psychological issues, but you don't want to overlook any physical cause. A change in a child's eating pattern is often a symptom of depression. Consider it in the context of your grandchild's overall behavior: Is there also a change in sleeping pattern? Is the child becoming withdrawn and isolated? If so, you may want to have her evaluated for depression and treated accordingly.

Children who hoard, like Eric and Daryl, need to be reassured that there is plenty of food. They do well with a consistent eating routine. If they know they will have breakfast, lunch, an after-school snack, and dinner at the same time each day, they can start to view meals as something they can count on. If they can tell time, they can see when the next meal will be. Children who eat too fast or too much may need to be monitored for a while. They should be served small portions and encouraged to ask for more if they are still hungry. You might also consider keeping healthy snack foods in a place your grandchildren can reach; this practice will reassure them that if they do get hungry, they can do something about it. It gives them a safe sense of control over their food.

A child like Joey has a different problem. For him, food is a way to manipulate Grandma. Why should he make an effort to eat by himself when refusing to eat earns him Charlotte's undivided attention? If you have a grandchild like Joey, understand that this is a different control issue: It is not about controlling food, it is about controlling you and the environment. If your grandchild can get you to sit in the kitchen for three hours trying to get him to eat, he wins. You can, however, step outside of the power struggle.

Again, the key is firmness, consistency, and patience. Have regular meals that last a usual and reasonable length of time. Let your grandchild know that if she hasn't eaten by the end of the meal, she may have to wait until the next one. Since children have a poor sense of time, it's a good idea to use a timer to let her know when the meal is over. When she realizes she won't have someone sitting and coaxing her to eat—and she misses a meal or two—she'll start eating.

If you do use this technique, you must be consistent. It doesn't do any good if you feel sorry for your grandchild and provide a snack later on. All he will learn is that he can eat whenever, and whatever, he wants. What you can do is remind the child that he can't have a snack today because he didn't eat his dinner, that perhaps if he eats dinner tomorrow, he can also have dessert. Don't forget to check with your pediatrician regarding vitamins and proper nutrients, and, again, make sure the problem isn't medical.

However your grandchild relates to food, don't ever withhold meals as punishment; eating should be a safe and reliable experience for a child, not something to be earned.

Babyish Behavior

Three-year-old Savannah reverts to using diapers and a bottle whenever she sees her mother, although she doesn't use either in nursery school or at home. "I think she thinks Mary wants her to be in diapers and bottles," says her grandmother, who traces Savannah's babyish behavior to the birth of her twin sisters. Ever since that time, Savannah has been possessive of her mother, trying to prevent her from holding the infants.

When young children feel threatened, they may revert to babyish behavior: thumb-sucking, baby talk, using a bottle, bed-wetting, clinging, wanting to be carried, or waking up in the middle of the night. A new sibling is certainly a threat. A child may feel insecure because everyone is paying attention to the baby in the family, a position she held until now. She may feel rejected if Mom keeps the new child but doesn't take her. A sibling is not the only threat a child faces; each time she sees a parent leave, it can feel like rejection. If her mother was nurturing during the child's infancy, an insecure six-year-old, hoping to bring Mom back, might revert to babyish behavior.

Understand that these are normal reactions. Most children will regress briefly, and need to, in order to work through changes in their life circumstances. Acting like a baby may be a sign that they need extra nurturing or need to adopt the role of a baby for a while. Eventually, they return to their more mature selves. Some children, however, will cling to this baby identity and not progress to the next stage of development.

If your grandchild is regressing, allow him some room to be a baby and work out the feelings. If the situation doesn't resolve itself, don't let it continue too long. You can address the insecurities without encouraging the babyish behaviors. You can validate the child's feelings with questions like "Do you wish you were still a baby?" or "Do you wish you still had your bottle?" Recognizing and understanding the feelings is different from encouraging the actions. You can reassure your grandchild that you love him and that he is very special but also remind him that he is no longer a baby. You can point out the advantages of being big and the disadvantages of being a baby: Big children can play with toys and watch television; babies take lots of naps and don't get to make decisions. Remind your grandchild to use words, not baby talk. Be reassuring and nurturing but also firm.

One more thing you can do is create a "life book" for your grandchild, that is, a collection of photos from the past arranged in chronological order, like a story, with descriptions underneath each photo. It is important for children to have a sense of roots and progress, and photos clearly document the passage of time. Your grandchild can see herself when she really was little, and she can see how much she has grown. There is a healing power in being able to hold your history in your hand and look at it, even for a small child. If you want to do a life book for your grandchild and you don't have access to early photos, start with the pictures you have. Add to the life book as often as you can, depending on your time and circumstances. You don't have to wait for major events like birthdays and holidays to take snapshots. Everyday activities can make charming photos and tell a story about a child's life.

Wanting to Call You Mom and Dad

A child who has a relationship with his parents already knows them as Mom and Dad and knows you as Grandma and Grandpa. Other children, however, may want to call you Mom and Dad; all the other kids have mothers and fathers, and your grandchildren don't like feeling different. Older children may even want to have their names changed whereas little ones tend to call anyone who nurtures them "Momma."

The truth is that you will probably have a harder time with this issue than your grandchildren. You may not want the children to forget their parents and may fear that this could erase their memory.

You might feel like you are usurping their parents' place. Or you might just be uncomfortable: You were a parent, now you are a grandparent, and you want the difference to be clear. When the subject of names comes up, don't make it a big emotional issue for a child. It is all individual, and there are no right or wrong answers. Whatever you and your grandchild are comfortable with will probably work fine. If you and your spouse are not comfortable being called Mom and Dad, you can tell your grandchildren that you are doing all the things a parent does but that they still have a mom and a dad and you are Grandma and Grandpa.

"Stuart asks me about how I can be both Grandma and Momma," says Arlene Townsend. "I tell him, 'I am what you want me to be.'" Three-year-old Tamara refused to call her mother "Mommy" when she saw her on visits. Her grandmother asked her why. "Her not my mommy," the little girl replied, "She's just my friend. You're my mommy. You take care of me every day." And Denise, who has lived with her grandparents from the day she was born, has it all squared away: Her grandmother is Grandma, her grandfather is Daddy, her Aunt Carla is Momma, and her mother is Momma Gail.

Tests and Manipulation

All children test limits; it is how they discover the boundaries in their world. They mouth off and act out and then learn from our reactions what is acceptable behavior and what is not. They don't fight fair, either. Children know just what to say, and when to say it, to get you to melt. They use scraped knees and hurt feelings, pouts, whines, and tears to get their way. Some parents handle the tests and manipulations of childhood better than others, but it is all part and parcel of raising kids.

Many grandparents forget this fact. Perhaps you haven't lived with small children in years and have allowed your memories of childrearing to mellow over time. You may be surprised and frustrated when your grandchildren are hard to handle; unfortunately, your grandchildren may be harder to handle than most children their age.

Tragic circumstances have given many grandchildren a distorted sense of limits. If parents were unstable and inconsistent—punishing today behavior they permitted yesterday—your grandchildren may see rules as flexible and changeable. Children who had free reign with their parents may have learned that they can do as they please. They may not think your rules apply to them and may resent your attempts to impose structure on their lives. They will test and retest the limits you set for them, beyond the point where other children would give up. Because these grandchildren struggle with profound feelings of rejection, abandonment, and poor self-esteem, they will also test how far they can go before you, too, reject them. They will push you away before you push them away.

Your grandchildren also have a stronger arsenal than most kids in the "I'm so unhappy; just do it my way" phase of childhood. While the reality of being neglected, abandoned, or abused is tragically painful, it may also be used as a means of manipulating adults. Every child cries "I want my mommy" when someone else—even Daddy—sets limits. (And if Mommy sets limits, "I want my daddy" might do just fine.) But it's a whole new ball of wax when it's a grandchild raised by grandparents. When Mommy might be in jail, on the streets, or even dead, a plaintive "I want my mommy" can just about kill Grandma, and she usually melts.

Don't underestimate the intelligence of children, particularly these kids. Many of them have picked up traits and characteristics from parents who are equally manipulative—addicts are the greatest con artists in the world—but most of these children are smart enough to push your buttons. They play for sympathy. They get Grandma and Grandpa fighting and take advantage of that. They tell their tragic stories to teachers, counselors, and peers as justification for poor behavior or as a means to get their way. When Kevin was in school, he once tried to get himself out of trouble by telling the teacher his mom had died. I think he believed he wouldn't have to be responsible for his behavior if he came up with something tragic.

Meanwhile, you start the game with your defenses weakened. Your grief at the situation, the split in your identity between grandparent and parent, your need to nurture these children and show them they are loved—all these factors make you vulnerable to manipulative behavior. There is, after all, a fine line between being a doting grandparent and a second-time parent with a need to discipline. Often you slip from one role to another almost without noticing it, and the kids know how to get you to do just that.

▪ HOW TO COPE

▪ *Set a clear, daily routine.* Children need consistency, particularly children who have suffered from loss and uncertainty. Try to make some aspects of your daily life predictable. Have clear expectations for each day, and warn your grandchildren about any expected changes. Recognize that change may trigger a repeat of unwanted behavior.

▪ *Offer positive choices.* Build regular choices into your grandchild's life. Allow him to have control over which book he reads at night, what stuffed animal he takes to bed, whether he eats his peas or potatoes first at dinner, whether he wears the blue pants or the green ones to school. Let him make decisions about things that don't matter to you or between two equally acceptable choices. Making decisions will give your grandchild a sense of control and may spare him from needing to seek power in negative ways.

▪ *State rules in the positive.* Whenever possible, tell your grandchildren what you want them to do instead of what you don't want them to do. You don't want to sound like you're constantly criticizing. If children follow positive rules, they feel they are accomplishing something, instead of simply succeeding in avoiding punishment.

▪ *Set limits and stick to them.* Children need firm, consistent limits. As much as they resist them, limits give children a sense of security and help them know what the expectations are in the world around them.

▪ *Present a united front.* Divide and conquer is a classic military maneuver, but kids seem to have an instinct for it. Your grandchildren know whom to go to for whatever they want, and they will play one grandparent against the other to get it. Try to make parenting decisions with your spouse, and stick to them. Otherwise, your grandchild may "win," and your marriage may suffer.

▪ *Learn to recognize manipulation.* One of the biggest problems in handling manipulative behavior is recognizing it, particularly in such troubled children. These children are surviving enormous tragedies, and yet some are arch manipulators. How do you know whether your grandchild is really missing her mother right now or just trying to stay up for another hour (or both, as is often the case)? You will need to rely on your instincts, the advice of counselors, and how well you know this child. Consider these factors: the timing of the outburst, the age of the child, and the child's level of sophistication. Put yourself in the child's place. Why is she doing this? If you have just refused to give the child a candy bar or it is bedtime, she may be trying to push your buttons. It's different when a child scrapes a knee and can't stop crying because Mom, who is no longer here, was most nurturing at such a time.

▪ *Separate feelings and actions.* Whether a child's tears or bid for sympathy stem from manipulation, emotional turmoil, or a combination of the two, there is one important thing to keep in mind: Feelings and behavior are not the same. It is important to reassure your grandchild that all his feelings are valid. He has a right to be sad or mad or upset. But, you can explain, feelings are not an excuse for not following directions or doing what is expected of him. You can certainly say, "I understand that you miss your mom. I miss her, too, and we'll discuss that in a few minutes, but it doesn't mean you're not going to bed on time." Likewise, children will say "You don't love me" as a way of diverting a situation. If it's time to make your bed: "You don't love me." If it's time to go to school: "You don't love me." "That's not the issue," you can tell them. "The issue is that you have to make your bed now because we're getting ready to go to school." Of course, always reassure your grandchildren that you love them. Children can't hear "I love you" too much. They just can't use it to get their own way.

▪ *Try to stay calm.* Sometimes children will push every single button you have, and you won't feel like being nurturing or loving. If you can, stay cool and collected. If you let your grandchildren realize they can get to you, you lose. Once they know they can shake you, it will be an uphill battle to regain control. Also, your grandchildren look to you for security and a sense of order. If you lose your temper, you may just confirm their conviction that all adults, like their parents, are out of control. This doesn't mean that you can't admit fear or sadness or anger, but children need to know that they can trust your stability.

OVERCOMPENSATION

Henrietta Casper has a problem. Her 15-year-old grandson is defiant and disrespectful. When she tells him he can't go out at night, he just walks out the door. Her husband would set firmer rules, but Henrietta can't stick to them. She promised her daughter on her deathbed that she would always care for Adam, and she can't find it in herself even to withhold privileges from the boy. Henrietta is falling into a classic grandparenting trap: overcompensation. She is trying to make up for the pain and the loss her grandchild has suffered by attempting to make him happy every moment, in other words, by always giving him what he wants.

It's an easy trap to fall into. Up until now you have been a grandparent and only a grandparent. You could dote, pamper, spoil, and comfort to your heart's content. It is hard to realize that you are now a surrogate parent and must also discipline and educate your grandchildren. It can take time for this new reality to sink in. Some grandparents can spend years caught between roles; they stay indulgent grandparents, rarely letting a day go by without buying something, however small, for their grandchildren. Then they don't understand why they can't get respect as parents. If you let your grandchildren have french fries and ice cream for breakfast, as one grandma did, it's hard to make them eat vegetables at dinner. You can't spoil them and educate them at the same time; you only send them mixed messages.

Grandparents who overcompensate do so materially and emotionally. Not only do they try to soothe their grandchildren with presents and surprises, but they overlook setting limits. They make allowances they never would have made with their own children. For instance, one day my mother told Kevin that he couldn't watch television until he made his bed. An hour later, I found Kevin in front of the television, and my mother was making his bed. She never would have done that with us.

It is important to realize that overcompensation doesn't help a child in the long run. No matter how much you do for your grandchildren, you cannot remove the pain, repair the loss, or fill the void that is inside them. The world has taken away more than you can put back. Nor do you do your grandchildren any favors by giving in. Children need limits to know they are loved and to develop a sense of who they are. All overcompensating does is teach them to expect permissiveness; it lets them feel that the world owes them things and that they don't have to behave or work to have them. Your grandchildren need to deal with their losses in the best way they can, with support and guidance from you and the other adults in their lives. They need a combination of nurturing and discipline, and they need consistency in both. They need to know that you will do what you say you will do, even when they may not like the outcome.

You can't make up for your grandchildren's past, but with time and patience you can build a foundation of trust, love, and security in the present. Real parenting doesn't bring the immediate smiles and laughter that presents do—sometimes it brings sour looks and loud complaints —but remember that you are doing more than making your grandchildren happy in the moment. You are giving these children the necessary tools to grow and build their futures.

PARENTING 101

Beth Grafton had already raised seven children of her own, so she was insulted when the judge who granted her custody of her grandchildren sent her and her husband to parenting classes. He was, she discovered, a prudent man. "We have been sentenced back 30 to 40 years in time," says Beth when she talks about parenting today. "We have to go back to our skills of the '50s . . . in the '90s!" And, she discovered, those years do make a difference. Grandparents who become surrogate parents are often ill equipped for the job. Childrearing has changed since you raised your own children, as has the society in which you raised them. Like Beth, you may find yourself trying to use '50s skills on children of the '90s, many of whom seem to know more than their grandparents.

Children have changed. Through television and other media, this generation knows more about sex, violence, and the world around them and at an earlier age than their parents did. And if your grandchildren came from a drug-using or abusive home, they may know even more about the adult world than other kids their age. The threats of drugs, gangs, and AIDS, combined with peer pressure, create additional parenting problems you weren't faced with 30 or 40 years ago.

Standards have also changed. Many disciplinary actions you may have used in the past are no longer accepted as parenting techniques. In fact, some are considered abusive. Francis Morgan, like many parents of the old school, used a belt to discipline her own children when they were small; today that could be grounds for removing a child from her home.

Some grandparents are shy of parenting. They feel they made mistakes with their own children and don't want to repeat them with their grandchildren. Others have been away from childrearing so long that they have forgotten how kids behave. They don't have a clear perspective on what is acceptable behavior and what should be disciplined.

Like Beth Grafton's judge, I recommend that grandparents look into parenting classes. You will find them offered through child guidance clinics, family service agencies, hospitals, and even local colleges. It's not that you are necessarily doing anything wrong with your grandchildren, but parenting classes can teach you new methods for helping them learn responsibility, accountability, confidence, and self-esteem.

Grandparent support groups are also a good resource. Grandparents who have taken classes are often happy to share their new knowledge with others in the group, and you may hear techniques you haven't tried. Perhaps your group could persuade a child psychologist to hold a parenting seminar specifically for grandparents.

If you don't have access to groups or classes, you can avail yourself of the good parenting books on the market. Moreover, popular magazines like *Parenting* and *Working Mother* regularly run articles about common childrearing problems and innovative solutions.

What follows is a brief list of the principles and techniques that might be taught today in Parenting 101:

- *Beware of physical punishment.* There is a fine line between discipline and abuse in handling children, a fine line between evoking respect and fear. Today, hitting a child with anything other than a hand on clothing may be construed as child abuse. I don't ever advocate spanking children. When you hit children, you teach them that anger and aggression are acceptable ways to solve problems. You teach fear instead of respect. It is much better for children to learn that actions have consequences. That kind of lesson lays the groundwork for better decision making as they grow older.

- *Reinforce good behavior.* Your grandchildren know that bad behavior will get your attention. And that is often what they want, regardless of how they get it. Therefore, the best way to create good behavior is to *pay attention to it*—with praise and rewards. Try to catch your grandchildren in the act of being good. Be specific in your praise; let them know exactly what behavior you like. Tell them that you see they are making an effort. Behavior charts and chore charts let children keep track of the good things they've done and give them a way to measure their progress toward a reward: an allowance, an ice-cream cone, a special day at the park with Grandpa.

- *Try time-out.* If your grandchild does misbehave, one of the more popular techniques in modern parenting is the use of a time-out. This resembles the old scenario of a child sitting in a corner, but it is meant more as a calming technique than as a punishment.

Time-out involves removing a disruptive child from the situation in which he is misbehaving and giving him time to cool off. It doesn't have to be a long time, just long enough to give him time to think about his actions. The actual amount of time will depend on the age of the child—more than two minutes is an eternity for a two-year-old, for example—but use a timer so that he knows that the length of time is not arbitrary. When the child returns to the situation, make sure he understands which behavior warranted the time-out. Communication is important in any discipline technique.

▪ *Make your consequences logical and appropriate.* The goal of discipline is to teach children to regulate themselves, to make them responsible for their actions. Discipline works best when you can link the punishment to the behavior. If a child throws food on the wall, she must clean it up (even if you have to do it again after she goes go to bed). If she insists on wearing shoes that are too small, let her wear them. If they hurt, she won't wear them tomorrow. Of course, allowing children to learn from their own mistakes doesn't apply in situations that affect their safety or anyone else's.

▪ *Make consequences immediate.* Children, particularly young ones, have short memories and a poor sense of time. They may not remember why they can't watch television tonight if they are being disciplined for something they did in the morning. Try to make consequences as immediate as possible; it makes them more effective and teaches the concept of cause and effect.

▪ *Reinforce cause and effect.* Children also have short attention spans. For any punishment or discipline to be effective, the child must connect the cause and the effect. For instance, if you give Susie a time-out for throwing sand in her brother's face, she may need help connecting the two events. Therefore, ask her at the end of the time-out why it was used. If she can say, "Because I threw sand at Tommy instead of using my words," she will not only remember why she was disciplined but will learn responsibility for her actions. The same principle applies with older children when you take away phone or bicycle privileges.

▪ *Teach responsibility.* Children do many things to test your reactions; they also do things they don't know are wrong. Sometimes it's worth letting one misbehavior go in order to teach responsibility. For instance, if John throws food at the wall, it doesn't hurt to give him another chance, provided he understands that if he does it again, he won't get to finish dinner, he'll have to clean up the mess, or he'll have a time-out. If again he throws food at the wall, he does it knowing what will happen. Again, discipline involves teaching children to regulate themselves; that means letting them make choices and take responsibility for the consequences.

• *Don't make empty threats.* It is never a good idea to threaten children; simply teach them that there are consequences to their behavior. If Joan doesn't do her chores, she can't watch television. If Mark hits his brother, he may have to spend time alone in his room. But make sure that the consequences are those that you, as the voice of authority, can follow through with. Grandparents have a particularly hard time setting limits and holding to them. You feel bad, you want to be nice, you give in. Thus, you end up teaching the children that they can get whatever they want if they make you feel bad. "No television for a month" is a great threat—but an empty one if you can't keep it. Withhold television privileges for the week, or even the night, and the children will learn that their actions have consequences. (Besides, if you do ban television for a month, you may be punishing yourself as well.)

• *Pick your battles.* Not every misbehavior is cause for confrontation. Some things can be calmly diverted and others simply ignored. If Mary Anne is writing on the table, try giving her paper first. The problem may stop there. Did Todd leave the room cursing under his breath because you turned off the television? Try letting it go. If he is disrespectful to your face, you need to deal with it, but he is entitled to feel unhappy and resentful and to express his feelings to himself. If you make each and every improper action into a crisis, you'll only squander your energy and foster a terrible relationship with your grandchild. Weigh the pros and cons before you make an issue of something. Ask yourself, "What do I expect to gain and what do I want the child to learn from this?" Then pick your battles accordingly.

THE HYPERACTIVE GRANDCHILD

Jewell Baxter's grandsons are three and four years old, and they are out of control. They have put silverware down the toilet and painted the walls with toothpaste. They urinated in the furnace and flooded the kitchen floor when Grandpa fell asleep (the floor alone cost Jewell $750 to fix). "You can't leave them alone a second," she says. "You just can't fall asleep!" If Emily Petersen turns around for a second, four-year-old Amanda is down under the house or up in the attic. Emily isn't physically able to crawl around looking for her when she disappears and is terrified that the little girl will get seriously hurt. Six-year old Gregory can barely control himself in school. He is a smart child, but he cannot sit still long enough to complete his assignments. Now he has begun to kick and beat up other children. Even in GAP meetings he bounces off walls. "I'm going to hang that little boy!" says his grandmother in frustration.

Sound familiar? Then you could very well have a hyperactive child on your hands.

A large percentage of the grandchildren I see and hear about are hyperactive, part of a condition called *attention-deficit/hyperactivity disorder*, or ADHD (it's called *attention deficit disorder*, or ADD, when there is no hyperactivity involved).[4] ADHD affects up to five percent of children under 18, or approximately 1 in 20 kids.[5] *Time* magazine calls it "the most common behavior disorder in American children."[6] ADHD is believed to be a neurological condition caused by heredity, medical problems, or prenatal exposure to drugs and alcohol. The result is difficulty with attention, concentration, impulsiveness, and self-control.

Simply put, children with ADHD have trouble concentrating, completing a task, sitting still, and focusing. They are easily distracted, are disruptive, and may have poor relationships with other children. They have little impulse control, acting before they think about the consequences of their behavior. They may get themselves into dangerous situations and not know why or how they happened. They require constant supervision, which can be exhausting for grandparents who may not have the energy or patience they once had.

Children with ADHD may be bright and yet do poorly in school, which can lead to their believing they are failures or bad kids. Poor self-image and low self-esteem are deep issues with these children. They don't mean to drive you crazy; their bodies just seem to move faster than their brains. One little girl came crying to her grandmother after acting up in school one day. "I don't know why I did those things," she said. "I don't know what happens to me, because I didn't want to do them."

Of course, not every child who gets into trouble in school or has difficulty concentrating is hyperactive. Some children appear to be hyperactive when the problem is really an emotional disturbance or a learning disability. Sometimes a child can experience a combination of the three. On the other hand, many children with ADHD are not hyperactive but may still exhibit difficulties with attention and/or impulsive behavior (they are diagnosed as having ADD). As with any disability, the various symptoms of ADHD and ADD may range from mild to severe, depending on the individual child and even the specific situation (i.e., some children may exhibit more problems in school or social settings than at home).

If you suspect your grandchild has ADHD or ADD, have him or her evaluated by a well-trained professional—a child psychologist, child psychiatrist, or a pediatrician who has training and experience in this area. There is no simple test for ADHD; a true diagnosis is pieced together, like a puzzle, from a variety of elements, including family and medical histories, a physical exam, psychological testing, screening for learning disabilities, and interviews with the child's caregivers and teachers. You can start the evaluation process through the school or community mental health clinic; some states provide early intervention services for children as young as one or two years old (see Chapter 13). You can also have your grandchild assessed by a private doctor. Mental health clinics and parent or grandparent support groups are good sources of referrals. If your grandchild is positively diagnosed with ADHD (or ADD), he or she should be referred to a child psychiatrist or psychologist for treatment, which should include counseling and may involve medication.

Medication for ADHD

ADHD is a complex disorder. It is not easy to diagnose, and there are some disagreements about how to treat it. Perhaps one of the main issues under debate is the use of psychoactive drugs like Ritalin, a psychostimulant medication that is prescribed by doctors as treatment for clinically diagnosed hyperactive children. Other drugs that are commonly prescribed include Dexedrine and Cylert. Although these drugs are stimulants, they seem to have a calming effect on children with ADHD.

Proponents of Ritalin applaud its effectiveness in reducing restlessness and impulsive behavior and thus helping a child concentrate and focus. Properly prescribed, drugs like Ritalin have allowed a calmer existence for hyperactive children, their families, friends, and teachers and have enabled these children to improve their school and social performance and feel better about themselves.

Critics, however, feel that doctors may be overmedicating children and are concerned about the drug's side effects, which can range from moodiness and insomnia to abnormally rapid heartbeats, nervousness, and lack of appetite. Meanwhile, parents—and grandparents—of children with ADHD must work with their doctors to make informed decisions based on the individual child and his or her particular needs.

I am not, in general, an advocate of medicating children, but I have seen hyperactive kids do a complete turnaround with the right prescription and dosage. In fact, many people compare the effects of Ritalin to putting glasses on a nearsighted person; glasses don't change the physical makeup of the eye, but they do let everything come into focus. Like glasses, drugs like Ritalin can be a tool, not a

---

Could Your Grandchild Have ADHD?

If a number of the following symptoms describe your grandchild, particularly if they started before age seven, and if they have lasted at least six months, you may have reason to suspect ADHD or ADD. However, a definite diagnosis requires a full examination by a qualified doctor.[7]

- Has difficulty concentrating
- Shifts excessively from one activity to another
- Often does not seem to listen
- Has difficulty following instructions
- Often fails to finish things he or she starts
- Has difficulty organizing
- Often loses things
- Is easily distracted
- Is frequently forgetful
- Fidgets or squirms excessively
- Has difficulty staying seated
- Has difficulty playing quietly
- Often blurts out answers to questions
- Often acts before thinking
- Often talks excessively
- Has difficulty waiting
- Often engages in dangerous activities

solution. However, finding the right medication and the proper dosage may take trial and error and patience. And not every child responds well to medication.

Talk to your grandchild's doctor carefully. Ask lots of questions. Consider all your options. Above all, if you do decide to use medication, make sure your grandchild is closely monitored by doctors on a regular basis. Look for any changes or reactions to the drugs. Try to involve teachers in the monitoring process as well; they will notice changes in school that you might not see at home. Make sure the treatment program is a well-rounded one. Medication alone will not cause long term changes. Nor will it cure depression or anxiety. Your grandchild also needs a combination of therapy and behavior modification to internalize and learn to use new behaviors.

WHEN YOUR GRANDCHILD NEEDS THERAPY

My own feeling is that most children who are taken in by grandparents could use some kind of counseling to handle the adjustment. Most could benefit from therapy, even as a preventive measure. Groups are great because each child realizes that he or she is not the only one with disturbing feelings. Most of these kids have such terrible self-esteem that even short-term therapy can help them understand that none of this is their fault. Children who act out their frustrations will often come to the attention of the school, which may then refer them to counseling. Unfortunately, the children who don't act out—the quiet ones or the good students—may slip through the cracks.

Does your grandchild need therapy? Counseling is especially important if any of the following statements describe your grandchild.

- The child has been physically or sexually abused.
- The child begins to remember past abuse. Sometimes you know the child was abused; sometimes this information only becomes available when something triggers the memories and a flood of painful emotions is released.
- The child seems depressed, particularly if he or she has been abused. (Remember, even very young children get depressed; observe your grandchild closely.)
- The child has been exhibiting behavioral, psychological, emotional, medical, or academic problems for a noticeable or prolonged period of time.

- The child is experiencing extreme fear or extreme anger.
- The child is sexually acting out.
- The child is constantly fighting or exhibits cruel behavior. (Often, kids who have been abused will then abuse their siblings, peers, and pets.)
- The child exhibits a combination of bed-wetting, fire-setting, and cruelty to animals.
- The child becomes self-destructive, talks about hurting himself or shows hints of wanting to die. People think young children don't think about wanting to die, but they do. The danger signs include any potentially self-destructive behavior, from walking out in front of cars to expressing thoughts of feeling unloved or saying, "I wish I weren't here." A child who lives with you because of a death may talk about wanting to be with Mom or Dad in heaven. Behavior like this is always a cry for help. Even if your grandchild uses it as a tool to manipulate you—and if he knows it gets to you, he could use it that way—it still masks deeper issues and needs to be dealt with in counseling.

RESIDENTIAL PLACEMENT

Seven-year-old Matthew had witnessed the murder of his father by his mother and was becoming dangerously aggressive in school and at home; on one occasion he tried to smother his younger sister. Nine-year-old Jesse had been physically and sexually abused before he came to live with his grandparents; he later started to act out sexually with his younger siblings. Sally, 10, is rebellious. She refuses to listen to her grandmother and repeatedly disappears from school and home. One night she cut the window screen and slipped out of the house with her grandmother's car keys, which she gave to a stranger who then stole the car; she didn't reappear until 1:00 A.M. and would not say where she had been. Six-year-old Nicholas is destructive. He tears plaster off walls and throws things at his grandmother. He was born with drugs in his system and is severely hyperactive. He, too, would sneak out of the house at night for hours.

Unfortunately, some children need more help than a grandparent can give them. They lack the ability to express their pain in words, and their actions put them and others in jeopardy. Some, like Matthew and Jesse, have experienced such deep trauma that they cannot control their behavior. Others, like Nicholas, are driven by chemical and neurological problems. Medication for hyperactivity, weekly outpatient therapy, and a grandma's love are not enough for these children. They need the more intense therapy that a residential program can offer.

A residential program is a live-in facility where children can receive round-the-clock professional care. A social worker or school psychologist often makes the recommendation to place a child in residential treatment, but grandparents can also request placement through the proper channels. Sally's grandmother, for instance, called child protective services and told them that her granddaughter was placing herself in danger and that she, as an ailing 80-year-old, could no longer handle her. Matthew, on the other hand, was placed through the department of mental health, after a school evaluation found him to be severely emotionally disturbed.

Children who are placed through child protective services or social services become dependents of the court, and their grandparents lose control over what happens to them. This is not so for children, like Matthew, who enter residential facilities through other channels; their grandparents may retain some control over their welfare even while they are in placement.

Giving up your grandchild to a treatment center is not an easy decision to make. It practically tore Nicholas's grandmother apart. "I look at Nicholas sleeping, and I cry," she admits. "But he is getting bad. Nicholas cannot help himself, and I don't have the knowledge to help him help himself." Nor is placement always a grandparent's decision. Sometimes grandparents don't recognize that they can't provide the home or guidance a severely disturbed child needs; in these cases the social worker may recommend placement over the grandparent's objections.

Placement, for any child, is an absolute last resort. No grandparent wants to put a grandchild in a facility, but if you have done everything in your power to help a child, and if she needs more than you can provide or is a danger to herself and others, residential placement may be your only choice. It doesn't mean that you don't love your grandchild or that you are abandoning her. You can still maintain contact through letters, phone calls, and visits. What it does mean is that you are giving the child her best chance to become a healthy, happy, productive adult.

GRATITUDE VERSUS GROWTH

Children are very self-centered; they have a tough time looking outside themselves. This is particularly true of children who have suffered loss. You may want them to be grateful for your hard work and sacrifices, but it is unreasonable to expect gratitude from a child who has been traumatized and who is angry about the situation. As adults they might look back and appreciate what you did for them, but right now they are just getting by.

It's ironic that the better the job you do parenting your grandchildren, the more likely you are to be taken for granted. Don't let it upset you. It means that your grandchildren have come to expect your love and attention and that it is not a rare treat in their lives. Take heart, instead, at the good you are doing.

Many grandchildren thrive under their grandparents' care— even those who were abandoned or abused. In fact, a 1992 study of 51 grandchildren being raised by grandparents found that the majority were making normal adjustments after living in their grandparents' home for an average of four years. A smaller follow-up study two years later surveyed the grandchildren's teachers for a second opinion. The teachers agreed: The children were still adjusting well. Although both studies were limited to children whose grandparents live above the poverty level and already attend support groups, researcher Michael Jones, Ph.D., believes his results give hope to all kinds of grandparents. According to Jones, it is the quality of the grandparent–grandchild relationship that is most important in a grandchild's adjustment.[8] "These kids are at high risk for emotional problems," he told the *Orange County Register.* "The fact that they aren't suffering those problems shows how resilient kids are. And what a good job a lot of grandparents are doing raising grandchildren."[9]

CHAPTER 7

Your Grandchild and the School

The hardest thing about school was adjusting with my friends. I really didn't understand my situation—how could they understand it?
—Kevin, age 19

J effrey Campos, age six, has a hard time set-tling down to his studies. Alternately shutting down and acting out, easily stimulated and hy-peractive, he can't function well in large classrooms. "Grandma, I can't stand the noise," he confesses when he comes home. "There's too much noise—people talking all the time!" The teachers say Jeffrey is intelligent, but he gets frustrated and overwhelmed. "For a while he didn't want to go to school at all," says his grandmother. "He thought he was stupid and couldn't do what the other kids were doing."

Heather Pierce, 10, has trouble reading; although she is in the fourth grade, she reads at a second grade level. She loves books but feels "dumb and stupid" because other children do so much better than she does. For their part, the other kids make fun of Heather.

Schoolwork is not a problem for five-year-old Bobby Franklin, but the classroom is. That is where he takes out most of his frustra-tion, by acting out and fighting with other children. Generally, Bobby is an average kid in terms of behavior—sometimes he listens, some-times he doesn't—but after he has had a visit with his mother, he becomes a minor terror in school.

School is rough for any kid. They get hassled about what they wear, they're expected to act a certain way, and they feel foolish if they're too different. And that's just with the other children. Strict teachers, rules and regulations, and the challenge of schoolwork itself can add new levels of stress to a child's life. But for a child being raised by grandparents, especially for a child with emotional or academic difficulties, school can be a minefield of problems, from social isolation to failing a grade.

BEING DIFFERENT: ODD CHILD OUT

Most children want to fit in, whether it is to the group playing hop-scotch on the sidewalk or to the class on a school picnic. Children raised by grandparents suffer the stigma of being raised in a family that is different. And other children can be cruel about differences. Not only do they seem to have radar to seek them out, but their playground teasing can be merciless. Fourteen-year-old Tyler re-members attending a parochial school in Boston where everyone knew that he lived with his grandmother, that his mother was an addict, and that his father was dead. The teasing was mean. The other kids cursed his mother and called her foul names; they said that his father killed himself because of Tyler and that his mom took off because he was ugly. Tyler admits, "The part that got me was they said my mom left me because she didn't really want me."

Adults face peer pressure in the workplace, children find it in the school yard. Even innocent childhood jokes can take on different, and painful, meanings for children who are surviving a loss. "I'm a little more sensitive to certain things than most of my friends," says my nephew Kevin. "When I got to middle school, people would rag on each other, just with friends. It was nothing serious, but they would start telling momma jokes, and stuff like that. I would take it personally, even though I knew they were joking around." The same kind of jokes started at least one fight in high school. "I don't remem-ber what the kid said," Kevin admits. "It didn't matter what he had said . . . just that he had said it."

Not only do your grandchild's peers make insensitive comments about the fact that you are older than their parents, but most school activities presume a parent–child relationship: from making Mother's and Father's Day cards to parent–teacher conferences. This can be troubling for the child who doesn't have a mother or doesn't know where she is.

BEHAVIOR PROBLEMS IN SCHOOL

All the emotional and behavioral problems your grandchildren experience at home may be exacerbated when they start school, and new ones may become apparent. Anxiety, fear of abandonment, and clingy behavior may take on new dimensions in a school setting. Your grandchildren face hours of not knowing where you are, how you are, and if you are coming back. Just taking them to school can be a trial if they are afraid you won't pick them up again. Some children even develop phantom health problems so you'll come and take them home.

Nor are school personnel always understanding. Ten-year-old Kirsten was tense and anxious after her grandmother had bypass surgery. Every time she heard an ambulance pass the school, she panicked. All day she asked if she could call home, just to make sure her grandma was fine, but the teachers refused her requests, believing that Kirsten was using the situation to manipulate them.

Anger, aggression, and inappropriate behavior may also find new outlets, and new triggers, in school. A little boy who has trouble with authority may defy his teachers. A little girl who is verbally or physically aggressive at home may hit or swear at other children. Your grandchildren may be bossy and have trouble making and keeping friends, which may only make them angrier. Many grandchildren only know how to get negative attention. They know how to push the buttons of their teachers and peers, just as they know how to push yours. They may get labeled as problem children, or acquire a reputation as poor students. They may skip school. Some may even fail and have to repeat grades.

On the other hand, withdrawn, depressed children may become introspective and shy at school. They seem to disappear in class. Their attitude is this: "If I sit in the back of the room and don't open my mouth, I won't get in trouble because they won't know I'm here." These children often get lost in the cracks. Loner kids may be viewed by teachers as a relief, as one less problem child to deal with. They may get good grades, but they may also slip by with Cs and Ds because they don't cause trouble; unfortunately, they may not learn anything, either.

New behavior problems in grandchildren may also appear in a classroom setting: difficulty following directions, difficulty playing with other children, difficulty waiting their turn. Many of the characteristics of attention-deficit/hyperactivity disorder (ADHD) and learning disabilities only come to the surface once a child starts school.

ADHD IN THE CLASSROOM AND SCHOOL YARD

As I mentioned in Chapter 6, many of the grandchildren I see and hear about have attention-deficit/hyperactivity disorder, which means they have trouble with attention and concentration; may be easily distracted, restless, or hyperactive; and are given to impulsive behavior. Although all children are inattentive, impulsive, and overly active from time to time, children with ADHD seem to be that way most of the time. For them such behavior is the rule, not the exception.

Children with ADHD face many challenges in school. They may have a hard time adapting to the classroom setting, performing their schoolwork, and acquiring the social skills necessary to make friends and play in groups. Children who have trouble with attention may have a hard time following directions or finishing projects. Long reading assignments and tests may be particularly difficult. If they are not hyperactive, they may be inattentive and underactive, appearing to daydream or wander off. They may be labeled "lazy" or "spacey" and accused of not trying. If they are hyperactive, they may be disruptive in class, constantly moving and unable to stay in their seats. Like Jeffrey Campos, they may be easily overstimulated and overwhelmed by a large, noisy classroom. If they are impulsive, they will act without thinking, calling out in class or blurting out answers before the questions are asked.

These traits may carry over to the playground, where children typically hone their social skills. A child with ADHD may interrupt other children's games or make jokes at the wrong moment. He may not be able to wait his turn, or he may frustrate easily and overreact. His behavior can lead to difficulty making friends, which can lower his self-esteem.

Each child with ADHD will demonstrate different symptoms and in different intensities, but the result will be a disorganized approach to learning and developing and a difficult time keeping pace with children his age. These children are not stupid. In fact, you may hear this remark from teachers: "Your grandchild! He is smart enough to do the work, if he would only *try*." It is not a question of intelligence but of attention and self-control. An informed teacher may recognize these behaviors as symptoms of ADHD. Unfortunately, an uninformed teacher may blame the child.

LEARNING DISABILITIES:
THE INTERNAL STUMBLING BLOCKS

April Thomas was miserable in grade school. Reading assignments took forever, classes seemed to rush by too fast, and tests were a nightmare. She would look at words on the blackboard and not realize she was reading them backward. She would struggle with a book and come away with only bits and pieces of the story. She would listen to her teacher's instructions but not exactly understand what was required of her. Some teachers got impatient with her many questions, so she stopped asking. "I would sit in class and pretend I understood what the teacher was saying," April, now 20, recalls. "Most of the time I didn't, but I was too embarrassed to admit it."

Because she was a bright girl, April was accused of "playing dumb" and of not trying hard enough. She was actually trying very hard, but it was a struggle to understand the questions, let alone come up with answers. Eventually, April got frustrated and gave up. She didn't want to seem stupid, so she became rebellious, making wisecracks in class. And she fell further and further behind her peers.

In high school April was finally diagnosed with learning disabilities. She received a tutor, special classes, extended time to take tests and turn in papers, and other modifications. Today she is a sophomore in college. April has learned to compensate for her learning problems and to enlist the help of teachers and administrators when she needs more time for assignments or permission to tape a lecture. Still, she is shy about her disability. "It's extra embarrassing because it is an invisible disability," she says. "If I had one leg shorter than the other and couldn't run fast, it would be a reason that people could see."

People may not be able to see April's disabilities, but many other children would understand them. Approximately five to ten percent of people are affected by learning disabilities, and nearly five percent of all school-age children receive special education services to help them compensate for different problems.[1]

Children who have learning disabilities may experience problems with reading comprehension, spoken language, writing and spelling, arithmetic, reasoning, and organizational skills. They may also exhibit symptoms of ADHD. In fact, many learning disabled kids also have ADHD. Like children with ADHD, learning disabled children are not dumb. They do not lack intelligence or a desire to learn. They have a problem with how they interpret outside information, a deficit in the psychological mechanisms that process selective visual, auditory, or tactile data. Learning disabilities must not be confused with problems due to mental retardation, serious emotional disturbance, or sensory deficits like blindness or deafness, which fall into other categories of disabilities.

Just because your grandchild has trouble with math or spelling, however, does not mean she has a learning disability. Many people experience learning *difficulties*—certain subjects they don't take to easily; there are, for example, children who love reading but hate science or who just don't seem to have a head for numbers. However, if your grandchild's problems are so constant or severe that they disrupt her education or day-to-day activities (such as reading street signs or using the telephone) or if there is a significant gap between the child's academic potential and academic achievement that is not the result of environmental, cultural, or economic disadvantage, then you may suspect a learning disability.

MISSED SCHOOL DAYS AND OTHER EDUCATIONAL HAZARDS

Not every child who has problems in school has ADHD or a learning disability. Your grandson may be behind in school simply because he missed too many school days before he came to live with you. Perhaps he was constantly on the move and changing schools with his parents. Perhaps drugs were involved, and getting a child ready for school wasn't the parent's priority. Your grandchild could arrive at a new school a grade or two behind, unable to read, and convinced he is stupid. He may also resist your insistence on regular school attendance, since he never had to attend school regularly before. Here, again, routine and consistency may start to correct the problem.

Another reason a child may do badly is worry. Your granddaughter may display a lack of attention in class because she is thinking about her parents and her circumstances. It can be difficult to complete class assignments, even to listen to the teacher, when a child feels the weight of the world on her shoulders.

Of course, difficulty with schoolwork could also be an indicator of a medical problem. Maybe Tommy does badly in school because he can't see the blackboard or has trouble hearing the teacher. Glasses or a hearing aid could be the answer.

■ HOW TO COPE

▪ *Talk to the teachers.* Whether your grandchild is hyperactive, acting out, or grieving, I recommend creating open lines of communication with the school. Talk to the teachers, counselors, and the principal; give them insight into your situation. Let them know that if your granddaughter misbehaves when she comes to class on Monday, there may be a reason. Explain that if she had a visit with a parent on the weekend, she is probably reeling with emotions, not simply being obnoxious. Often teachers are more understanding if they know there is an explanation behind a child's problem behavior.

If his teacher understands that Johnny lives with his grandparents and doesn't know where his mother is, she might be more sensitive to his reaction to making a Mother's Day card in class. Maybe she'll have the children make cards for "someone who is special" instead, since not all children live with their mothers or fathers. Having a teacher recognize such a circumstance may give it authority in a child's eyes, and that recognition may soften the stigma of not having a parent to make a card for. The nuclear family of a mom, a dad and their child is something we can no longer take for granted. Sensitive teachers, being aware of this, have learned to reference grandparents, aunts, uncles, foster parents, and adoptive parents in their lessons or comments about family, family events, and family history.

Your grandchild's teacher may also be your ally in identifying symptoms of ADHD or a learning disability, since some traits may only appear once a child is in school. If you suspect that your grandchild has a developmental or learning problem, share your concerns with the teachers and start to compare notes. If your grandchild does have ADHD or a learning disability, ask what you can do at home to help the child progress.

Of course, many teachers are overwhelmed. They may have 40 kids in a small classroom, each with different problems, and might not be able to give out special help or consideration. Still, the more you can communicate with the teacher, principal, or school counselor, the more your grandchildren will learn about problem solving. If they are children of substance abusers, they have already learned a lot about running away from problems; this is a chance for them to learn that problems can also be worked out. I have on occasion recommended moving a child to a different classroom, but only as a last resort and never before exhausting all other possibilities.

▪ *Talk to the child.* Jeffrey's grandmother tries to reassure him before tests. "You know it," she tells him. "Just listen and think about what the teacher is asking you, and you're going to be fine. Just do the best you can; we can't ask for more than that." Heather's grandmother tries to keep her from comparing herself to other children. Your own attitudes about learning and the way you communicate them to your grandchildren can influence the way they approach the school experience.

Talk to your grandchildren. Help them emphasize and develop their strengths. Maybe your grandson has trouble with math but is good at basketball, singing, or drawing. Praise him for what he does well, and create opportunities for him to succeed. Every success will boost his self-esteem and encourage him to strive for more success. And teach him to understand his weaknesses. You can reassure him that everyone has some kind of difficulty and that there is no shame in asking for help. Remind him that everyone learns at a different pace and that having difficulty in a subject doesn't mean that he is stupid or dumb or bad. At the same time, don't be so easy on him that you give him permission to give up. His situation may create particular challenges for him in school, but it is not an excuse for him to stop trying. Tell him that he may have to work harder but that he can succeed. Encourage him to keep doing his best. Still, keep your own expectations realistic. If your grandson really does his best, you cannot ask for more.

▪ *Look into special education.* Just because some children are currently trailing behind the rest of the class does not mean they are doomed to stay behind. Free special education and related services are available to children who are somehow handicapped in the learning process. If there is a chronic problem that prevents your grandchild's schoolwork from matching her intellectual ability, whether it is a learning disability, severe emotional turmoil, or a physical handicap, the child should be eligible for special help through the school system. In fact, most states offer special services to disabled or potentially disabled children before they even enter the school system (see "Start Early," below).

The process of applying for special education will help you and your grandchild uncover the source of her academic troubles and, hopefully, find the solutions. Sometimes the solution is as simple as obtaining a hearing aid, therapy, or a tutor. It was discovered through testing that one little girl who was doing poorly in school was actually gifted; her poor grades were due to boredom and a lack of confidence.

If your grandchild is having consistent problems in school, try to address them as soon as possible. At least start documenting what you see, and if the situation continues to worsen, request an Individual Education Program, or IEP (see Chapter 13).

• *Start early.* It is never too early to consider your grandchild's development and learning potential. Children who experience educational and developmental difficulties are often overlooked until they fall severely behind their classmates. By that time, their academic performance has already suffered and they may feel depressed, anxious, and inadequate about school.

You do not have to wait until your grandchild starts school to get the benefits of special education. Physical therapy, speech and language remediation, and other services are often available to children before they even enter kindergarten. Most states offer early intervention programs that are designed to address developmental problems in the preschool years, when children are typically most ready to learn—and at an incredible pace. These are preventive programs that assume that the earlier children get help, the more chance they have of succeeding later.

If you notice in your grandchild the absence of anything typical for a particular stage of a child's development or any delay in motor coordination, speech, or self-help skills like self-feeding—or if drug exposure or family history have you concerned that problems could develop—look into an early intervention program. Some states even provide services to infants and toddlers. (For more on early intervention, see Chapter 13.)

• *Seek out peer activities.* There is more to a child's school years than simply sitting in a classroom. Extracurricular and recreational experiences are as important for developing social skills as a good education is for developing learning skills. Your grandchild may have taken on many caretaking responsibilities at an early age and may not know how to be just a kid. Scouting organizations, after-school clubs, summer camps, day camps and athletics provide opportunities for children to *play* with other children and learn to socialize, share, and take turns. Extracurricular activities involving sports, arts, and music also offer children who have academic problems a chance to discover other strengths and build a sense of self-esteem.

▪ *Find young role models.* Children, particularly those who don't have parents as role models, desperately need the influence of young adults. A younger person may have more energy and stamina than a grandparent. He or she may more clearly understand the choices and challenges a child faces growing up today than can older grandparents whose ideas may seem old-fashioned. My nephew Kevin often points out that his grandparents were "brought up in the old days, like in the time of World War II" (that can seem like ancient history to a child growing up in the '80s and '90s). Even kids who have youthful, active grandparents can benefit from the influence of younger adults.

Extended family can be a wonderful source of role models for a grandchild, and many grandparents successfully involve aunts and uncles in their grandchildren's lives. In my family, for example, my brother was the one who would play ball with our nephew Kevin and take him to sporting events. Beth Grafton's son and daughter-in-law take her grandchildren on vacations. However, not every grandchild has extended family members available. Some aunts and uncles may be caught up with their own families or may live far away, or they may disapprove of your raising the child and therefore keep their distance. Even if the parents were only children, you can still find young adults to interact with your grandchildren. Big Brother and Big Sister programs exist across the country to provide positive role models for children who need them. I know one little girl whose Big Sister continues to visit her even in a residential facility. Scouting programs, summer camps, and youth groups also bring together children and active young adults, as well as provide fun activities and new experiences for the children.

▪ *Aim high!* Don't let academic delays or learning disabilities stifle your hopes for your grandchildren. History is full of disabled people who succeeded in the face of tremendous challenges, and many people with learning disabilities have gone on to become scientists, lawyers, generals, even president. Consider the following examples:

> Albert Einstein didn't talk until he was four or read until he was nine; he couldn't learn math through traditional teaching

methods. His first teachers thought he was backward. Yet he grew up to win the Nobel Prize in physics and to revolutionize the way we think about space and time.

Young George Patton couldn't read or write by age 12. Still, he overcame his disabilities enough to be appointed to the U.S. Military Academy at West Point; he went on to become a general and led the Third Army in Europe during World War II.

Woodrow Wilson had learning problems as a boy. He was 8 years old before he learned his letters and 11 by the time he learned to read. His relatives considered him "dull and backwards." The only school subject he excelled in was speech. Yet he grew up to become the 28th president of the United States.[2]

Is your grandchild a future Einstein, Patton, or Woodrow Wilson? No one can really say. One of the wonders with children is that we don't know what they may become. So help them aim high. The possibilities are all ahead of them.

CHAPTER 8

The Drug Epidemic at Home

Our young people—the young parents—are
dead because so many of them are hooked on
crack. The grandparents are trying to save the
little ones before the same thing happens to
them.

—Marin County social worker[1]

Jim and Fay Strassburger have watched an entire middle-class neighborhood lose child after
child to drugs. They can stand in their yard
and point to the houses. In one week in the early '70s, they attended
three funerals for kids who died of drug-related causes, bright kids
who knew the consequences of their actions. Their own son and
daughter are alive but struggling with drug and alcohol addiction; two
grandchildren live with Jim and Fay. "We've lost a whole generation,"
Jim told a reporter. "Maybe part of the next."[2]

Katherine Connor is raising five drug-exposed grandchildren, all
from the same daughter. She can frequently be seen doing her er-
rands with the infant tucked under her arm and the rest of the children
trailing after her like a line of small ducks. The mother is on the
streets and often violent. She once threw a brick through the kitchen
window, almost hitting her own son with a piece of broken glass.
When she was picked up by the police, she broke the windows and
the grill of the police car—that's how much violent strength she had
from PCP.

There is no question that we are in the midst of a national, even
an international, drug epidemic. The nightly news is full of stories
about local gangs, foreign drug lords, and the victims of drug-related

crime. But there are other victims: infants exposed to drugs before birth, young children abused and neglected by drug-abusing parents, and grandparents who turn their lives upside down to keep their families together. In the war against drugs, the front line is often at home.

Drug addiction and alcoholism are not new problems in our society. The 19th century had its morphine addicts.[3] Marijuana and LSD reached new levels of popularity in the 1960s,[4] and by the 1970s babies were being born exposed to heroin and PCP.[5] But in the mid-1980s the smokable form of cocaine powder, known as crack, first appeared in the United States, and America's drug problems intensified.[6]

Crack is a relatively cheap, fast high that is more addictive than heroin or cocaine used nasally. Unlike heroin and other drugs that have traditionally appealed mostly to men, crack is used increasingly by women,[7] many of whom are pregnant or of childbearing age. According to *Time* magazine, crack has "lured far more women into addiction than any other hard drug has."[8] It has also triggered the use of other drugs: heroin, to prolong the cocaine high, and tranquilizers and alcohol, to "come down." The result is a growing population of young people addicted to multiple drugs and infants exposed to a wide variety of drugs in the womb. Crack is also a mean drug, inducing many parents to violence. There has been a dramatic rise in reports of child abuse and neglect since the 1980s, the majority of them traceable to parental drug and alcohol addiction. In one five-year period, child abuse reports tripled in the state of Wisconsin alone.[9]

The rise of AIDS has added another frightening dimension to the drug epidemic. "AIDS is now the largest killer among young women [here]," said an East Coast health official. "We may not have to worry about [crack baby] mothers; they'll all be dead."[10]

Meanwhile, the next drug crisis has already arrived in the form of "crank" or "ice." Crank is a metamphetamine derivative that speeds up the nervous system.[11] It is more expensive than crack, but it offers its users a longer high. It is also known to produce extensive fetal damage.

These facts read like horror stories, particularly to grandparents who helplessly watch their sons and daughters sink into the terrifying reality of addiction and then try to pick up the pieces of their families. For these grandparents home is the battleground against an enemy they barely understand, and the only weapons they have are love and knowledge.

This chapter looks at some of the things you need to know in your own private war on drugs: the truth about addicts and addiction; the symptoms, risks, and needs of drug-exposed children; and suggestions for stopping the cycle of addiction in your grandchildren. Appendix A includes a list of organizations that can provide more detailed information and guidance. Remember, this is a difficult fight, and addiction is a fierce enemy; you can only take each day, and each battle, as it comes.

ABOUT THE ADDICT

There is no way to count how many addicts there are in this country. Some statistics say that 20 million Americans have tried cocaine at least once, that 5 million use it on a regular basis, [12] and that six times as many people abuse alcohol as use cocaine. [13] But those numbers don't necessarily account for the people who regularly use and abuse marijuana, heroin, PCP, or even legal prescription drugs. It probably doesn't matter. For a family struggling with the effects of addiction, even one addict is one too many.

I know grandparents who have spent thousands of dollars and all their energy trying to get their adult children into rehabilitation programs only to see them relapse and return to the streets. They witness the thoughtless abuse and neglect of their grandchildren and are often helpless to protect them. They spend sleepless nights asking the questions: "Where is my child?" "When will he recover?" "Doesn't she see what she's doing to us, to her children, to herself?" "How can we help him?" "Where did we go wrong?" If your adult child is an addict, these questions are probably not strangers to you. But before you can really answer them, you must first understand what addiction is and what it does to the addict.

What Addiction Is

Chemical dependency is not a moral weakness, bad habit, mental illness, or sign of weak character. [14] It is not a result of life's pressures or a temporary loss of control. Addiction is a disease characterized by a mental and physical dependence on a chemical substance. A person becomes chemically dependent, or addicted, when he or she develops a craving for a substance as a shortcut to feeling pleasure or avoiding pain, including the pain or discomfort of not using the substance itself.

Like many diseases, addiction is chronic, that is, it is constant and long-lasting. Addiction is also progressive in that it gets worse and worse over time, requiring more and more of the substance to achieve the good feelings and prevent the bad ones. And, for some addicts, it can be fatal.

High hopes, good intentions, and promises will not cure the disease of addiction. Intense rehabilitation, strong support, and—for some addicts—medical attention are necessary to bring an addiction under control. Few addictions are truly "cured."

What Addiction Does

Addiction takes over the addict's priorities and makes his behavior unpredictable. The high that originally seduced him gets harder and harder to achieve. It becomes the most important thing in his life—more important than family, friends, work, food, sex, anything. An addict may spend every waking hour trying to get or stay high. The disease can lie to him, making him forget the bad things that happen—the lows, the pain of withdrawal, the effects on his family. As one drug counselor put it, "If there are drugs behind you, your own son will run you over to get to them."[15] One social worker compared counseling an addict to "beating your head against a brick wall . . . because you are dealing with someone who has no control over her life. She's worried about her next hit."[16] Some young mothers have sold their baby's milk and diapers for drug money. Others sell their bodies, supporting their drug habit by becoming street prostitutes. As one former addict explained to a U.S. Senate committee, "Even though I wanted to quit, my need for the cocaine was greater than my maternal instinct."[17]

Addiction can also stunt a person's development. Pam Marshall sees it in her daughter. "It's frightening what it does to them," she says. "Once they start using the drug, they stop growing intellectually. Linda started using at 13, and her mind is still like a 13-year-old's. It's like she lost all the years in between." Another grandmother describes her adult son as "24 going on 14."

The behavior of an addict is controlled by drugs and alcohol. His behavior doesn't mean that your son doesn't love his children; her actions don't mean that your daughter is trying to hurt you. If your adult child doesn't seem at all like the child you raised, she probably isn't: drugs and alcohol have taken over her life.

■ WHAT YOU NEED TO KNOW

▪ *It's not your fault.* Pam Marshall remembers trying to explain her daughter's addiction to herself. "It was my fault," she says. "It was her father's fault. It was her peers' fault. You blame everyone and everything except the person herself. You look for excuses. You look back and try to figure out what happened, when it happened, how it happened . . . and you don't have any answers." There is no one answer for why a person drinks or takes drugs or why one person will become an addict and another one will not. But you are not to blame. You could raise four children and have only one of them turn to drugs. You could be an alcoholic yourself yet raise a family of staunch nondrinkers. Though you may never have touched a drop of wine, your child may be an alcoholic. We each make our own choices in life. Your children made theirs.

▪ *There is little you can do to help.* One of the most frustrating things for parents to accept is the fact that there is nothing they can do to *cure* their child of a drug or alcohol addiction. Remember, an addiction is a disease. You can't make it go away. Nor can you make your addicted child seek help. Certainly, you can drive your child to a treatment center or support group, but he is the one who must enter, stay, and participate. Too many parents pay for treatment after treatment when they are the ones who are motivated, not the addict.

If you want to facilitate treatment for your adult child, you can give her a list of programs in your area. You can watch her children while she is in rehabilitation. But if she is not ready to make her own appointment and show up for treatment, then it will only be an exercise in futility. The addict must be the one to recognize the problem and commit to seeking help.

All you can do is protect yourself and your grandchildren and try not to give in to your adult child's pleas and demands. An addict will use you, and you have to understand that. If you give addicted child money, you finance his habit. You have to be strong enough both to love your child and to refuse him. It is the old rule of tough love (for more on tough love, see Chapter 5).

▪ *Recovery can be painfully slow.* Recovery from an alcohol or drug addiction is a long, complex process with no guaranteed results. Many people don't complete treatment programs, and the relapse rate is high. Even when addicts successfully complete a program, they are still at risk for returning to old habits. And they often can't tell you what happened or why. In 1991, several grandparent families from GAP appeared on *Donahue.*[18] Two of them were accompanied by their adult daughters, each of whom was in recovery and doing well. Unfortunately, a year later both daughters were back on the street. One was back in jail, where she gave birth to her fourth child.

Crack addicts relapse more than other drug users. According to one expert estimate, only 25 percent of crack addicts will remain drug-free for six months after treatment, compared with 50 percent for chronic alcoholics and 60 percent for heroin addicts in a methadone maintenance program.[19] "The statistics for recovery are a lot like the statistics for weight loss programs," says Jacqueline Battle of the Infants of Substance Abusing Mothers clinic at Los Angeles County–University of Southern California Medical Center. "How many people a year later have gained it back?"[20] Thus, getting into treatment is an important start, but there is still a long, frustrating fight ahead.

▪ *Seek emotional support.* If you have an adult child who is an addict, find a source of information and support. Al-Anon and Nar-Anon are 12-step groups for people who have relatives addicted to alcohol and drugs. Physicians, mental health professionals, and substance abuse counselors can help you understand what is happening to your child, and grandparent support groups can give you a forum where you can express feelings and frustrations and receive reassurance that your feelings and concerns are normal. Don't try to weather your child's addiction alone; find a source of emotional support and use it often.

▪ *Give up hope* . . . It sounds strange to say, but sometimes the kindest thing you can do for yourself is to give up hope. Hope keeps you paying for treatment after treatment, looking for the magic one. Hope keeps you and your grandchildren waiting at the door imagining that this time Mom or Dad will be sober and committed to abstinence. The truth is that your son or daughter may—or may not—recover. But the battle is not yours. You cannot make your child better; it is not in your control.

▪ . . . *but expect anything.* Despite all the doom and gloom predictions, some people do recover. Something in them is resilient enough to fight back and win. Sometimes the most unlikely candidate for success will surprise you. Take the story of Dorsey Nunn, a prisoners' rights advocate in San Francisco. A recovered addict himself, he took in his nephews when his mother died. "I'm sure Mom didn't recognize when I was serving a life sentence that I'd be the one raising the family," says Nunn. "You can look for hope in the most unlikely circumstances. Besides, if no one advocates for recovery, grandparents will be raising grandchildren for a long time to come."[21]

YOUR DRUG-EXPOSED GRANDCHILDREN

Katherine Connor hardly slept at all the first five months after her third granddaughter arrived. Because the drug-exposed baby had a tendency to stop breathing at night, Katherine slept at the foot of her own bed, propped high on pillows so she could look down into the crib. Her clothes laid out nearby, Grandma was ready to run to the hospital if she had to. As Becky got older, Katherine finally got to sleep for intervals of three to four hours.

Baby Jay was also born with drugs in his system. He could barely breathe, his body was unusually rigid, and the doctors thought he might never walk. When she first saw him, says his grandmother, "He was frantic. His little eyes darted from side to side. His tongue came out like a serpent's tongue. You knew he had problems." When he first came home from the hospital, Jay went through four months of "withdrawal," shaking and crying uncontrollably. One weekend he screamed for 52 hours straight. Sometimes his grandparents would float him in warm water to calm him down; then they would swaddle him tight in a blanket and rock him through it.

Pam Marshall feels lucky. Although her daughter Linda was a 20-year addict, her granddaughter Megan was born free of drugs in her system. "My miracle baby," Pam calls her. Still, she doesn't know what could happen 10 years down the line. There is too little information about the long-term effects of prenatal drug exposure for Pam to feel completely safe that Megan is in the clear, and she continues to watch her granddaughter closely.

Some studies estimate that one in every ten newborns is exposed in the womb to one or more illicit drugs[22] (one in five in major cities like New York and Los Angeles).[23] However, because many private and suburban hospitals do not routinely test pregnant women or newborns for the presence of drugs in their system[24] and because even positive toxicology screens only identify drug use within the previous 24 to 48 hours,[25] no one really knows how many children were exposed to drugs and alcohol during uterine development.

Whatever the statistics, the result of a pregnant woman's addiction can be heartrending: an underweight infant, shaking and crying; an underdeveloped toddler; an older child who shows a range of difficulties from learning disabilities to emotional and behavioral problems. For grandparents, unprepared to raise a second family, drug-exposed children are an exhausting challenge.

The following paragraphs discuss what you need to know about drug-exposed children: the symptoms and risks of prenatal drug exposure on children; the special demands on you as caregivers (e.g., the late-night vigils ahead of you); and recommendations from experts and other grandparents on how to handle common issues like tremors and uncontrollable crying. Understand, however, that no one can present an exact picture of how a drug-exposed child will look or act. There is no formula, no equation, to guide you. Much depends on what substances the mother took, how much of them she took, and at what point in the pregnancy she took them.

Nor does every child react to drug exposure equally. Some children may exhibit many symptoms whereas others may not experience any. Some children may have difficulties that only appear as they get older. Although the outcome of prenatal drug exposure can vary from one infant to another, all babies born to substance-abusing mothers are at risk for developmental, learning, and behavioral problems, as well as for fragile physical health.

The symptoms and risks discussed in this chapter are only generalizations. They are not included to scare you but to keep you aware of the possibilities. Try not to look for trouble, but, at the same time, keep your eyes open for the small signs that suggest that your grandchild might require extra help. The earlier you catch problems, the sooner you can address them.

Is Your Grandbaby Drug Exposed?

It is easy to tell if your grandchild was exposed to drugs in the womb if the infant tests positive for unprescribed medication or drugs in his or her system at birth. Unfortunately, toxicology screens only show drug use within the previous 24-to-48-hour period. This means that a fetus can be exposed to drugs and alcohol for months before delivery and these substances will probably not show up in his or her system if the mother abstained from chemical abuse during the week before delivery. If that was the case with your grandchild, prenatal drug exposure is a puzzle you and your doctor must piece together from a variety of clues.

The following signs may indicate prenatal drug exposure in an infant if several are present and not due to some other medical condition.[26] If you suspect your grandchild was exposed to drugs in the womb, contact a physician.

- Premature birth
- Low birth weight
- Small head
- Seemingly constant shaking or trembling
- Difficulty feeding
- High-pitched, inconsolable cry
- Difficult to comfort
- Seizures
- Is unresponsive and lethargic
- Diarrhea
- Vomiting
- Frantic sucking
- Stiff, rigid body
- Staring or unusual eye movements
- Irregular breathing pattern
- Startle response to the least sound or touch
- Easily overstimulated
- Sleeps too much
- Doesn't sleep at all
- Physical signs of fetal alcohol syndrome (FAS), such as small, widely spaced eyes, small, flat cheeks, and a short, upturned nose

Drug-Exposed Infants

The first few days after delivery can be quite an ordeal for infants born with drugs present in their systems and for the people who care for them. The babies go through a process similar to chemical withdrawal, which can include tremors, seizures, and uncontrollable crying. They can be frustrating to care for, since they do not respond to many of the cues normal infants respond to, like bouncing and cooing (in fact, some will even arch their back to get away). The stress of this period means that a drug-exposed infant can miss out on some of the early weeks of learning and bonding, which are so important to a child's emotional development. Once any actual drugs are gone from the baby's system, there can still be physical and psychological ramifications from the prenatal drug exposure, as well as possible medical risks.

Drug-Exposed Toddlers and Children

Children of substance-abusing mothers are at risk for a number of challenges as they grow up. Respiratory and neurological problems, visual and hearing deficits, birth defects, cerebral palsy, and mental retardation are not uncommon in drug-exposed children, although not every such child will have medical complications. Some of these children may have difficulty with motor development; their hands may shake when they reach for objects and they could have trouble learning to walk. Some may be slow in learning to talk or in completing toilet training. They may be easily stimulated and may show an inclination toward hyperactive and impulsive behavior. They may have difficulty paying attention, which can cause problems when they start school. In fact, many drug-exposed children exhibit symptoms of attention-deficit/hyperactivity disorder (ADHD) and various learning disabilities. However, each of these conditions has been associated with many different outcomes. Whether a condition becomes a handicap or a challenge has a lot to do with how a child is helped and how his or her needs are met.

It is important to understand that the effect of drug exposure is unpredictable. There is no typical drug-exposed infant or child. Experts do not know exactly how much prenatal exposure will affect a child's development. Not all babies exposed to drugs and alcohol suffer equally. Some children may be obviously affected by their mother's addiction: Like Becky, they may be premature and medically fragile. Like Jay, they may suffer through symptoms of withdrawal. They may have the facial characteristics often associated with fetal alcohol syndrome. Some children may not seem to be affected at all; they may look and act just like other children, but learning and/or behavioral problems may show up in preschool or kindergarten. Others, surprisingly, may completely escape harm.

How an individual child is affected can depend on what the mother used and when in the pregnancy she used it. It can depend on her health and nutrition and on whether or not she received prenatal care. It can depend on the temperament of the individual child. It might also be a question of luck. We just don't know enough yet to predict. "It's like throwing dice," says Jacqueline Battle. "You really can't tell what will happen."[27]

But while substance abuse by the mother doesn't guarantee damage to the infant, all children born to substance-abusing mothers are *at risk* for problems as they grow up.

▪ HOW TO COPE

▪ *Reduce stimulation.* Many drug-exposed infants are easily stimulated and difficult to calm. This can be particularly troublesome when you're trying to get the child to sleep. If your grandchild is an overly excitable baby, consider reducing the outside stimulation in the environment. Try to eliminate loud noises, bright lights, sudden movements. This is hard to do with other children in the house, but do as much as you can. Consider what you have on the walls and in the crib. Is it bright and distracting? Can you keep lights low? Can you turn off the television? Speak to the baby in a soft voice, or hum and rock to soothe him. Don't handle or jiggle the baby too much, and try not to do too many things at once, even soothing things. It will just rev him up all over again.

▪ *Try swaddling.* Two of the symptoms of a drug-exposed infant are a prolonged, piercing cry and uncontrollable shaking. Unlike normal babies, who cry but eventually fall asleep, drug-exposed infants are unable to calm themselves and will continue to cry and shake and flail their arms and legs. Your first instinct might be to rock the baby or to pace with or bounce her up and down as you whisper soothing sounds. Unfortunately, these things only add to the stimulation. Try swaddling instead. Wrap her snugly in a blanket and hold her close to your body. Soothing the baby in this way cuts down on her own activity and reduces the stimulation. "You wrap them close to you and let them feel your heart," says Katherine Connor. "It's like kittens with a clock."

Never swaddle a baby who has a fever or trouble breathing.

▪ *Be vigilant.* Raising any child requires you to be constantly alert to signs of illness or sounds of trouble. Drug-exposed children demand twice as much vigilance, since they may be medically fragile as infants and hyperactive as toddlers. "You need to watch these babies during the night," says Alice Sutherland, a former pediatric nurse who is raising two drug-exposed grandchildren. "They have a lot of problems in the first years. You have to stay alert. You don't sleep soundly, or you're going to lose them. You need to monitor them and go into that room and actually feel them."

Once drug-exposed children start walking, the issues change. You can't assume that the child is still in bed or that the child gate is still keeping her out of danger. The question is not "How is the child?" but "Where is the child?" "These are not dumb children," says Alice. "You have to out-think them. When it's quiet, think, 'Why is it quiet?' And find them quickly."

▪ *Learn about these children.* If you know or suspect that your grandchild is drug-exposed, educate yourself. Talk to doctors, experts, and grandparents who have been where you are now. The more you know about the effects of drug exposure, the earlier you can address any difficulties your grandchild may have, whether they involve a hearing deficit, a language delay, or poor motor control. If you suspect any kind of problem, take preventive measures. Get your grandchild a thorough physical and look into early intervention programs.

▪ *Look into early intervention.* Every state offers early intervention programs to address developmental and learning disabilities before children enter the school system. Some states even provide services to infants and toddlers. If you think your grandchild could benefit from early intervention, contact your state board of education and ask which department handles such programs. (For more on early intervention, see Chapter 13.)

▪ *Find outside support.* A drug-exposed infant can make you feel like a failure. Many of the things you did to soothe and care for your own babies may not work with this one, and you may not know why. Still, many grandparents are reluctant to admit they don't know what they're doing and are shy about asking for help. Don't suffer in silence; look for support. The National Association for Perinatal Addiction Research and Education (NAPARE) provides free information on caring for drug-exposed children. Grandparent support groups are also a wonderful source of advice and support. Not only do they offer you a forum to express your frustration, but they are a place to hear other grandparents' experiences and the solutions they found. "Drug-exposed children don't come with instructions," says Jacqueline Battle. "No kids do."[28]

▪ *Avoid the dangers of labels.* For several years now, the media has reported on the tragic stories of "drug babies" and "crack babies," painting pictures of damaged infants who will never have a chance in life, who are "born to lose," as one headline put it.[29] But just because a child was exposed to drugs does not mean that he is doomed by them. Remember, the effects of drug exposure are unpredictable. Moreover, many of the symptoms that drug-exposed infants experience are similar to those of premature infants who were not exposed to drugs or alcohol in the womb.

The trouble with these labels, besides being unfair and inaccurate, is that they can limit our understanding of an individual child. If relatives, teachers, or physicians focus too closely on the fact that a child's mother was an addict, they run the danger of assuming that all the child's problems are caused by prenatal drugs and may not consider other possibilities, such as heredity, disease, or emotional distress. One baby kept returning to the hospital with what everyone thought were seizures; now the doctors believe he was suffering from frequent ear infections. Labels can also create self-fulfilling prophecies. If you expect a child to fail, he probably will.

If your grandchild was exposed to drugs in the womb, definitely watch for related symptoms. But watch for all kinds of symptoms—just as you would with any child. Don't let anyone dismiss your grandchild as a "drug child" without asking deeper questions.

▪ *Know your grandchild's family medical history.* As more and more medical conditions are proving to be hereditary, it is difficult to overemphasize the importance of a family medical history. Respiratory problems can certainly be related to drug exposure, but they can also be inherited. Hyperactivity is also believed to be a genetic condition. Poor feeding can be signs of an allergy to milk. The more you can find out about your grandchild's family background, the better you can help your pediatrician attend to the child's needs. Even if the child is placed with you from a foster home, ask for any available medical records or medical history.

▪ *Don't lose hope.* Prenatal drug exposure can be a serious medical and developmental challenge for a child, but it doesn't have to be a sentence to failure. The jury is still out on the long-term physical and psychological effects, and some early studies indicate that with proper intervention there is reason to hope for a good outcome in many cases. In fact, some experts predict that many children prenatally exposed to drugs and alcohol can develop into healthy children and responsible members of the community. "This is not a lost generation," says Dr. Evelyn Davis, a pediatrician at New York's Harlem Hospital. "These children are not monsters. They are salvageable, capable of loving, of making good attachments. Yes, they present problems that we have not dealt with before, but they can be taught."[30]

Alice Sutherland knows the truth of that statement. All three of her grandchildren were born drug exposed, and she has seen them make great strides in their development. When the oldest was struggling in public school, Alice put her in a magnet school for the performing arts, hoping the child's love of music would give her motivation. Sarah is still only an average student, but at age 13, she has already appeared in a television commercial and hopes to be an actress someday. "Success," says Alice, "all depends on the person raising the child. The drug is just a medical problem the first five or so years. Intellectually, these children are very intelligent. You watch; you'll see all individual people."

▪ *Love, love, love them.* Children learn to trust the world when they have consistent and responsive caregivers who accept them as they are and who provide them with a safe environment in which to strive. The more they trust their immediate world, the more they trust themselves to try new things. If there is any medicine that is guaranteed to work wonders on your grandchild, it is your love. It's the secret ingredient every grandmother knows:

> "You're going to have to know that your life stops on a dime," says Fay Strassburger. "The only thing that exists at that time is that baby, because that baby needs all the attention, all the love and all the caring you can possibly give him."[31]

"They thrive on that," says Alice Sutherland. "That's what gets them through—knowing they are secure and that there's a lot of love."

"This is love," says Katherine Connor. "That's the key to why my babies are all surviving; they know they have a grandma who loves them."

STOPPING THE CYCLE:
RAISING THE NEXT GENERATION

Jessica Hulsey, 15, is a crusader against drugs. The daughter of addicted parents, the California teenager knows firsthand what drugs do to a family and to a child, and has spoken out against them in compositions, school assemblies, and newspaper articles. "I missed a lot," she told the *Orange County Register*. "I grew up so fast, and I had to worry about my sister and family. I will never forgive drugs for taking [normal life] away from me."[32]

Although they may not be as vocal as Jessica, many children of addicted parents harbor intense negative feelings about drugs and alcohol. They have seen what it does, and they swear they want no part of it. It's the kind of statement that fills a grandparent's heart with relief. Unfortunately, however sweet they are, declarations and promises are not guarantees. Don't let them lull you into looking the other way. The sad fact is that children of alcohol and drug abusers run a high risk of using drugs and alcohol themselves, almost 10 times the risk that children of nonaddicted parents face.[33]

The combination of peer pressure and curiosity about drugs and alcohol can be overwhelming to teenagers and children. Your challenge, then, becomes how to prevent an at-risk grandchild from becoming an at-risk teenager. While there is no foolproof way to keep a child off drugs, there are some precautions you can take:

▪ *Accept the possibility.* "Not my child." Those are the three words that get a parent, or grandparent, into the most trouble when it comes to drugs and alcohol. They keep you from watching for changed or strange behavior, they keep you from asking questions and finding help, and they offer you false hope. The truth is that any child may bend to peer pressure and curiosity. The only way to stop the cycle of drug and alcohol abuse is to understand that it is a cycle and that your grandchild may be at risk for addictive behavior. Don't bury your head in the sand. If a grandchild's behavior seems suspicious, ask questions.

■ *Teach your grandchildren to say no to drugs.* If your grandchildren are old enough to understand, talk to them about drugs. If you have already discussed the subject in talking about their parents, continue the conversation. It is not enough to teach them to refuse drugs; they have to know why, and your best examples may be close to home. Provide them with clear, factual information. Look at your own use of alcohol and tobacco; what messages are you sending? Nurture your grandchildren's self-esteem, and discuss different ways of handling peer pressure. A child who is prepared to say no may have an easier time actually saying it.

■ *Supervise your grandchildren.* The best way to know what is happening in your grandchildren's lives is to be actively involved in them. Know their friends and their interests. Be aware of where they go and whom they're with. Don't allow your involvement in their lives to deteriorate into an inquisition but maintain it as a normal part of your relationship. Not only will you be aware of changes in their lives, but you may build a closer, more trusting relationship with them.

■ *Learn to recognize drug use.* Unlike childhood diseases like mumps and measles, drug abuse does not have overt physical symptoms. However, there are warning signs a grandparent can watch for, if you know enough to look. They are the same signs many grandparents innocently tossed off as "growing pains," "teenage changes," and "the flu" when they were raising their own children: changes in eating and sleeping patterns, restlessness, sudden sulking or excessive energy. The accompanying box lists the symptoms of teen drug use. Familiarize yourself with them and stay active in your grandchild's life; if the changes are there, you will then be in the best position to spot them.

Don't be paranoid, however. It can be difficult to know the difference between erratic but normal behavior in kids and behavior caused by drugs. Every change is not an alarm. The changes to be concerned about are those that seem severe or that last more than a few days. Even if they are not linked to drug use, changes could signal medical problems, depression, or trouble at home or at school. If you do suspect anything, seek professional help.

■ *Seek outside help.* Drug information alone may not be enough to keep a child off drugs. Self-esteem, positive role models, and peer

Could Your Grandchild Be Using Drugs or Alcohol?

The Warning Signs

Although experimenting with drugs and alcohol has almost become a rite of passage with teenagers, many children don't limit themselves to curious experiments. Instead, they slip down the steep path to habit and addiction.

Has your grandchild:

- Become hostile or uncooperative?
- Become withdrawn and depressed?
- Suddenly dropped old friends?
- Become careless about his or her appearance?
- Lost interest in favorite hobbies or sports?

Is your grandchild:

- Suddenly doing poorly in school?
- Skipping classes?
- Experiencing unexplained bursts of energy?
- Experiencing a severe weight loss?
- Experiencing a change in eating or sleeping patterns?
- Unresponsive or aggressive with family members?

Does your grandchild seem:

- Constantly tired?
- Restless?
- Excessively talkative?
- Irrational?
- Drunk or spacey?

Many of these symptoms could be warning signs of excessive use of drugs or alcohol, as are dilated pupils, needle marks, and the presence of drug paraphernalia like needles, water pipes, pills, and roach clips.

Many of these symptoms are not limited to drug use; they can also indicate depression, an eating disorder, or some other psychological or medical problem. Whatever their cause, they warrant investigation.

support are also important. Many schools and youth groups sponsor antidrug programs. There are also a number of national organizations that can help you help your grandchild stay drug free: The National Institute on Drug Abuse (NIDA) runs a hotline that provides information, referrals, and emergency counseling. Mothers Against Drunk Drivers (MADD) has programs to help children develop positive self-esteem and refusal skills; the Boy Scouts of America sponsors antidrug campaigns and publishes a booklet for children; and Al-Anon runs support groups for the children of alcoholics called Alateen and Alatot. Check your yellow pages under *drug abuse* and *alcohol* for groups in your area.

A FINAL WORD

The information in this chapter has presented only some of the possible outcomes for drug-exposed children. Many of these outcomes can be frightening to consider, but they are only generalizations. They are designed to help you keep your eyes open, not to cause despair. Your grandchild's life is still being written. If anything will give them the chance to succeed, it is your love and patience in raising them.

CHAPTER 9

When Parents Get Their Children Back

What makes me scared is that my mom could take me anytime she wants. I always told myself if she does come and try to get me, I plan to run away. I'm not going to lead that hellish life.
—*Cameron, age 15*

Grandma's house was a safe house for Marjorie Brown's two grandchildren. Jessica, age three, arrived at the age of six months with fingernail marks up and down her back and a huge bruise on one leg. Her mother, Valerie, told Marjorie to take Jessica before she hurt her. Billy came almost a year later, when child protective services removed him from his mother because of neglect. Valerie, a drug addict who had been involved with gangs since she was 14, had been in and out of jail on several counts and had only seen Billy four times in eight months. She had not complied with court-ordered counseling or drug programs and was not allowed to see her children without another adult present. Even Valerie's parole officer described her as a "walking time bomb." When the unthinkable happened and a juvenile court judge decided Valerie was ready to parent and ordered Billy back to his mother, Marjorie was floored. In her wildest imaginings, she hadn't expected this. She knew Valerie couldn't handle the baby. The social worker knew it. Even Valerie knew she wasn't ready for full-time motherhood—and said so. However, the judge, noting that Valerie had had several clean drug tests and that she wanted unmonitored visits, decided she was ready.

Today, Marjorie and Valerie have a voluntary arrangement. Billy lives with Marjorie, but Valerie can take him whenever and wherever she likes. Marjorie is scared to death. She sees Valerie driving around with gang members and dressing like one; she worries that her daughter is using drugs again. She is afraid of drive-by shootings with the baby in the car. Mostly, she is afraid of her daughter's temper. "Billy's at the point where he's walking and getting into things," she says. "Valerie has already expressed that she couldn't handle him, and she'd only had him twenty-four hours. She couldn't take the stress of his screaming. I'm afraid she's going to hurt him. If she could hurt Jessica at six months, what could she do to Billy?"

In addition to her own fears, Marjorie is having problems with Jessica. Jessica's court case is separate from her brother's, and she is not legally affected by the judge's decision. Nevertheless, the emotional toll has been heavy on the little girl. She had begun to open up and play with other children; now she is withdrawn and is having nightmares. She sees her mother taking Billy, and she is terrified that she will have to go with her, too. "She wakes up in the night screaming, 'I don't want to go with Valerie!'" says Marjorie. "I hold her and tell her she is not going, but she sees Billy come and go, and she doesn't know what to make of it. She used to love to go to McDonald's. That's our meeting place now. She won't eat at McDonald's anymore. That's pretty bad, when a child doesn't want to eat at McDonald's."

Sending children back to their parents can be a grandparent's fondest dream—and worst nightmare. The dream is that the adult children will shape up and become active, responsible parents, that the grandchildren will be safe, and that you can resume your role of occasional baby-sitter and doting grandparent. The nightmare is that the children will go back before the parents have their lives in order, before it is truly safe.

For some grandparents, dreams do come true. There are parents who hit a bad patch in their lives and come out of it. There are addicts and alcoholics who recover and resume normal lives. Unfortunately, there are also many grandparents who wake up to discover the nightmares are real: A mother who hasn't seen a child in three years shows up and wants him back; an absent father remarries and suddenly wants his children; and the court decides that the parents are ready to take their children again, although, as far as the grandparents know, they are still using drugs. Nothing can prevent the shock and heartache of sending a child back to potentially unfit parents. Even when you know it can happen, you don't want to believe that it will. But when you don't see it coming, the pain is that much deeper.

FOREWARNED AND FOREARMED

The truth is that unless you have adopted your grandchildren or the parents are dead, you are at risk of losing them. If you have the children on an informal basis, the parents have every right to take them, even after several years. If they have been placed with you through the juvenile justice system, you should be aware that the court's goal is to reunify children with their parents and that everything will be done to accomplish that. Even if you have private legal guardianship, it can be overturned if the parents prove themselves fit (although this puts the burden on the parent and is less likely). Neither you nor your grandchild is protected from the parent's ultimate right to parent, and you need to be prepared for anything, particularly when you deal with the juvenile court. Knowing these facts won't lessen the pain if you lose your grandchildren, but it can help you prepare for the worst.

Remember, you may have little control over what happens to your grandchildren tomorrow, but you have a lot of control over what happens today. You can give your grandchildren the best care you can while you have them. You can give them a foundation of love and self-esteem. If they are old enough, you can teach them skills to take care of themselves—simple things like how to call 911, how to make a peanut butter sandwich, how to call you collect. One grandmother taught her twins her phone number by inventing a song. You can also make sure they know that certain kinds of spanking and touching are not okay and that they should talk to a trusted adult if anything like that ever happens, even while they are living with you.

IF THE UNIMAGINABLE HAPPENS

If you do have to give up your grandchildren, you will feel like your heart has been torn out. Your life will be turned upside down yet again. You had traveled the road from grandparent to parent; reorganized your life around these children; and loved and nurtured them for months, if not years, and now you will be expected to give them back like any part-time baby-sitter. It's hard, and it's painful. All the complex feelings you went through when your grandchildren first arrived double back on you with a vengeance. But now there are new layers: guilty thoughts that if you had handled something differently, they might still be with you; false hopes that maybe your adult child really can get it together this time; renewed rage at the system and the parents; uncertainty over if and when you will see your grandchildren again; fear for their safety; and a feeling of deep helplessness over your inability to protect them. It can feel like there is a huge void where your heart should be. You might find yourself distancing from them, if only to protect yourself.

Your grandchildren will have their own mixed reactions to going back to their parents. They may repeat behaviors that you thought were long behind them: bed-wetting, explosions of anger, school problems. Children who don't want to leave you may feel like you're sending them away; they may regress or push you away, or they may misbehave, hoping that if they're bad enough, their parents won't want them. Children who want to be with Mom or Dad may stop listening to you once they know they're going home. They, too, might misbehave, thinking that if you've had enough, you'll send them sooner. They may be caught between conflicting feelings and may express them in angry outbursts.

Either way, your grandchildren are being uprooted again and will need help with the transition. If you are lucky, you will have time to prepare them. You can reassure them that you are not sending them away and that you'll try to keep in contact. Although you can't speak for what Mom or Dad will allow—parents may lie to their children about allowing them to see you—you can promise your grandchildren that if you can't see them, you will think about them and continue to love them. Children who start acting out behaviorally will need help putting their feelings into words. If they are in counseling, they need to focus on this change. Also, let teachers know what is happening so that they can help, too.

Sometimes, however, you don't have the luxury of transition time. The judge in Marjorie's case would have let Mom take the baby directly from the courtroom, with no transition at all, except that Valerie herself objected. If this happens, all you can do is give yourself room to grieve.

If, like Marjorie, you have other grandchildren at home, you will also have to deal with their reactions: fear that they, too, might have to leave; anger at being left behind; sorrow at being separated from their siblings; or fear for their siblings and concern that they may never see them again. All you can do is reassure them that you love them, that you understand their feelings, and that for now they are safe with you. Unfortunately, it is the man in the robe who is making the decisions.

Then there are the practical issues. What do you send with the children? Do you give Mom all the baby's things? Certainly, you want the child to have them, but will that be the case? Or will Mom sell the high chair for drug money? And what if Mom can't parent two months from now and the kids come back to you? Won't you need a high chair and car seat? My recommendation is to play it by ear. Everything depends on your individual history with the parent. Do whatever you are comfortable doing. Perhaps you can give a few things at a time and see what happens. Look at the whole picture before you decide what, and how much, to give away.

OUT OF SIGHT, OUT OF REACH

Perhaps the hardest thing for a grandparent to face in this situation is the wrath of the parent who believes you "stole" the children (even if it was the juvenile justice system that removed them in the first place). Parent–grandparent relationships will be strained at best and can escalate to outright hostility. In the worst cases, parents deny grandparents all access to the grandchildren.

A Wisconsin grandmother had to spend close to $30,000 in attorney fees just to get one monthly visit and one weekly phone call with a granddaughter she raised for nine years. A Minnesota grandfather used to go to his grandsons' school to watch them play ball, but Mom got a restraining order so that he can't even do that anymore. These grandparents send cards and gifts without knowing if they are received. Some are returned. They have lost grandchildren not only from their homes but also from their lives.

▪ HOW TO COPE

When your grandchildren go back, it can feel like the world has ended and the nightmare has begun. Nothing will take the pain away, but there are some things you can do to help yourself adjust.

▪ *Give yourself time to grieve.* Your sadness, your anger, and the huge sense of emptiness are normal. You have suffered an enormous loss, and you need to process your feelings in a safe, comfortable way. This is a time to seek out support. If friends and family are too overwhelmed, consider counseling. And definitely seek out support groups. Just because you no longer have your grandchildren doesn't mean you are barred from grandparent groups. If anything, this is a time when you most need to be with people who understand the depth of your loss.

▪ *Try to move on.* It sounds cold, but there's not much you can do once a judge has decided that a parent is rehabilitated. Whatever is going to happen will happen. Perhaps the parent *has* pulled together. If not, maybe the child will end up back in the system and they'll call you. But you can't put your life on hold until then, and it won't help your grandchild if you do.

▪ *Get busy.* Spend time with your other grandchildren; they also need you in their lives. Volunteer. Some grandparents have found it helpful to volunteer in a hospital or a school when they miss being around kids. Get involved with all the hobbies you put on hold. Spend more time with people you care about—your spouse, family, and friends.

▪ *Get politically involved.* Many grandparents at the front of the grandparents' movement have channeled their grief and anger into activism. They may not be able to help their own grandchildren, they reason, but they can fight to prevent other grandchildren and grandparents from suffering similar traumas. One of the hardest things to accept as a grandparent is how helpless you are in the system; political action offers you a chance to affect the system and empower yourself in the process (see Chapter 15).

THE NEVER-ENDING CYCLE

Two of Sandra Cobb's seven grandchildren were returned to a mother who swore she was off drugs. She tested clean, met regularly with her probation officer, had a steady job, and appeared to be ready to care for two babies. It didn't last. Several months later, Mom resumed her drug use, lost her job, and started prostituting again. When she left the boys alone in her apartment, a neighbor called the police. The children were taken into protective custody and given back to Grandma.

When you are returning your grandchildren to their parents, it is cold comfort to think that they might soon be back. It means that they will have been mistreated again and that they will return to you with emotional wounds reopened. It is rare that children go home to Mom and Dad and actually stay with them. Another truth about these adult children is that they rarely pull it together for long. They go into rehab. They get jobs. They even stay clean for one or two years—long enough to impress a judge and raise your hopes. But they walk a thin line between good intentions and immediate gratification, and they are prone to misstep.

After years of self-protection, Pam and Robert Marshall finally allowed themselves some hope. Linda had been clean nearly two years. She had a job and an apartment. She started to show more than a passing interest in her daughter, calling and visiting more often, and she started talking about a future for herself. Then something snapped. She started using drugs again. She got pregnant and hooked up with an abusive ex-boyfriend whom she tracked down in jail. Now she's back in rehab, and her parents are devastated.

Even as you grieve the new loss of your grandchildren, brace yourself for anything. This, too, could be temporary. If you are allowed to see the children, keep a close eye on them. Try to stay on the parent's good side, even if it means walking on eggshells to do it. Offer to baby-sit. Above all, continue to document. Even if you are barred from seeing your grandchildren, keep a log. Whenever you make a call or send a card, even if the parent interferes with your attempt, write it down. If you can, find some way of knowing where your grandchildren are and how they are. If they are removed again—and they very well may be—you need to know about it.

SECTION II

Through the Red Tape

CHAPTER 10

Grandparenting and the Law

Never to such an extent in U.S. history has care
of children by relatives been so interwoven
with government.
*—Newsletter of the National Association
of Court-Appointed Special Advocates
for Children*

I f you are a grandparent raising a grandchild, the
odds are good that at some point you will end
up in a courtroom. The process could be as
simple as filing for guardianship with the parent's consent; it could
be as heartrending as a fight to keep your grandchild from being
returned to an abusive home. Either way, powerful strangers—
judges, social workers, and attorneys—will be able to determine
what happens to your family. Even if you are not raising grandchildren, you could find yourself rubbing shoulders with the law. The
divorce rate is approximately one out of every two marriages, and
some grandparents have to petition the courts just for the right to
see their grandchildren.

Many grandparents have gone their entire lives without entering
a court of law. They may think that law, like violence, is something
that happens to other people—those in the newspapers or on television. But they do believe in justice, and they expect it to be there
when they need it. Then they enter the legal system and discover
that justice is confusing, impersonal, and often outrageously expensive, both financially and emotionally. The cost can attack your bank
account and your spirit. The process is painfully slow. Moreover,
the underlying principles are not friendly to grandparents. As one

Texas grandmother told the *Katy Times*, "The courts treat you as though you're some old busybody who just doesn't like the way your kids are raising their kids. They act as though you have no right whatsoever to care about these babies."[2]

Although this book cannot change the attitude of the legal system, it can attempt to clear up some of the confusion. This chapter and the next are designed as road maps of the key legal issues you may encounter with your grandchildren, namely, your rights as a grandparent, possible custody arrangements, and the landmarks of the juvenile dependency system. They are designed to give you enough information to ask informed questions. Knowledge is power, and the best protection you have in any battlefield is an understanding of your opponent. First, however, a few warnings:

▪ *The legal system is complex and changeable.* It is couched in gray areas and interpretations, and the interpretations are as different as the judges who make them. To quote one family court judge, "I can't say, 'This is the law, and if you connect the five following dots, you win.'" Law is never that simple.

▪ *Family law is governed by state, not federal, legislation.* This means that laws and regulations about marriage, divorce, paternity, custody, visitation, guardianship, adoption, and foster care vary from state to state, as do the legal definitions of child abuse and neglect. What is called probate court in California is surrogate's court in New York. "Visitation" in one state may be "access" or "parental contact" somewhere else. "Guardianship" may be "managing conservatorship." I have used names that are either common or self-explanatory, but you may encounter different terms, laws, and regulations in your own state or county.

▪ *Grandparent issues are uncharted waters,* not only for grandparents but for attorneys, judges, and government agencies as well. A Chicago couple seeking custody of their grandson wrote that their attorney had been in practice for 28 years and had never handled a case like theirs before. The same may be true of the judges who hear these cases. Even child welfare laws were designed with nonrelated caregivers in mind. As one attorney put it, "State legislatures are ten years behind the social phenomenon."[3]

Your case will be shaped by the specific details of your situation, by the particular laws of your state, and by the bias of the judge who hears it. If you need legal advice, talk to an attorney who specializes in your specific area of law: family law, guardianship, child welfare, and so on. He or she can advise you on the basis of the facts and circumstances of your individual case.

YOUR RIGHTS AS A GRANDPARENT

"Grandparents have all the responsibilities and none of the rights," says Barbara Kirkland, founder of Grandparents Raising Grandchildren.[4] In many ways this is true. In our society grandparenthood is a biological connection, not a legal one. The laws and regulations that protect the family presume a nuclear unit of mother, father, and child. The grandparent–grandchild relationship can be severed by adoption, divorce, and even the whim of an angry parent. In fact, until recently, relatives had no greater access to a child than nonrelatives.

Today, however, almost every state has some kind of visitation statute that allows grandparents limited rights to request visits with their grandchildren (although the court can still refuse the request). This makes the right to petition for visitation the only legal right you have *as a grandparent*. In some states or counties you may also have certain privileges, such as first preference for placement if a child is removed from a parent's custody by the juvenile court system, but these privileges relate more to government policy about the child than to your rights as a grandparent or relative.

To understand your apparent lack of clout as a grandparent in America, you must understand the power of parents.

THE PROTECTED RIGHTS OF PARENTS

Traditionally, parents have had almost exclusive authority when it comes to their children. Our government cannot dictate how people raise their children, nor can it randomly take their children away from them. Unless a child is in some kind of danger, no one, not even the court, can interfere with the parent–child relationship. Even when a child is legally removed from a mother or father's care, every effort is made to enable him to return safely home.

The idea that children belong with their parents is at the very root of our social structure.

In theory, such airtight rights are a wonderful thing. There are countries where the government easily interferes with family relationships. Our country was created on the principle of broad individual rights, and the right to privacy is one of them. Imagine a social worker, lawyer, or relative being able to come into your house to tell you how to raise your own children, and you may see why parental rights are worth protecting. Unfortunately, in practice, the children are often the losers. The laws that favor parents presume that they are able to care for their children and keep them safe. The issue of children's rights is rarely addressed because until recently few people thought about children as having individual rights and it was assumed that any rights children did have would be protected by their parents. The exploding numbers of abused and abandoned children in recent years has proven that assumption to be painfully false.

Even when the state does intervene, the rights of the mother and father seem to overshadow the right of the child to be safe from harm. That is because the legal standard commonly used in custody and visitation cases is "the best interests of the child."[5] Yet there are no legal definitions of "best interests." Judges have a lot of discretion in deciding what it means.

This unshakable belief in parents' rights is the most powerful opponent you will encounter in the legal system. If you can understand that, you have a better chance of understanding and adjusting to the battles you may fight as you try to obtain custody of your grandchild.

THE LEGAL CUSTODY OF GRANDCHILDREN

Custody is one of the main problems facing grandparents who are raising grandchildren in their homes. Without custody, you may have problems enrolling a child in school, getting medical care, or seeking government aid. Without custody, you have no control over whether your grandchild is handed back to an abusive, neglectful, or intoxicated parent. Even with some kind of custody arrangement, your power may be limited.

Custody is confusing because people use one word to mean many things. A grandfather whose grandson lives with him may call it custody. A grandmother whose granddaughters were placed with her by the court may call that custody. Grandparents who have legal guardianship of their grandchild will say they have custody. And each does have a small piece of the custody puzzle.

Custody defines a relationship of control over and responsibility for a minor child.[6] There are two kinds of custody—physical and legal—and that is where the confusion lies. If a child lives with you, she is in your *physical* custody, but you may not have *legal* custody. Physical custody means physical control over a child, including the right to have her live with you. Legal custody means legal authority to make decisions about the medical, educational, health, and welfare needs of the child. These distinctions are common in divorce settlements, where the parents may have joint custody (shared legal and physical responsibility for a child) or one parent may have full custody (legal and physical) while the other has visitation rights. But divorce is not the only circumstance that puts the custody of a child in question. The legal system can transfer the custody of a child in order to protect her from danger. This is where grandparents come into the picture.

If your grandchild lives with you, the child is physically in your custody, whether you have an informal arrangement or a formal one. The more critical questions are these: Who has legal custody? What is your legal relationship to the grandchild in your care? What are the limitations of your arrangement?

There are four types of custody situations that may affect your grandchild; each has legal and financial consequences for your family. They are informal custody, court placement (and/or foster care), guardianship, and adoption. Another issue you may be involved with as a grandparent is visitation. While this is not a matter of custody, it affects many grandparents deeply.

Informal Custody

Many grandparents who have grandchildren living with them have no legal arrangements for doing so. They start out caring for the children on a casual basis and seem to continue that way. Some grandparents don't even realize that there are legal options available to them. This makes informal custody one of the most common arrangements among grandparents. With informal custody you have, in essence, physical custody of the child while legal custody remains with the parents. Unfortunately, this situation offers the least protection for you and your grandchildren.

Informal custody can mean constant struggles over school enrollment, medical care, and financial assistance. Many school districts may not allow a nonparent to enroll a child unless he is the legal guardian, and relatives can run into difficulties obtaining medical care for a minor child. One Texas grandmother had a notarized letter from her daughter authorizing her to seek medical attention for her grandchildren, and the doctor still refused to treat them. Although the Texas Family Code allows adult relatives to seek medical care for a child, the doctor has the right to refuse treatment if the adult is not the legal guardian.[7]

On the plus side, informal custody means you don't have high court costs and attorney fees or government interference with your family. But it also means that you are at the mercy of the child's parents; they can take the child whenever they want to, and you will have no legal means to stop them. You are, in fact, little more than a glorified baby-sitter. If you only have informal custody of your grandchildren, you have no real control over their safety. In fact, your desire to protect them makes you vulnerable to emotional and financial blackmail by their parents. As long as you are without legal protection, you are open to parental manipulation.

▪ HOW TO COPE

▪ *Look into government aid.* Just because you have informal custody of your grandchildren does not mean you must shoulder the financial burden alone. Your grandchildren may be entitled to financial and medical assistance through one of several government programs (see Chapter 12 for details).

▪ *Look into guardianship.* If your grandchildren are not in the custody of the juvenile justice system, you may be able to file for guardianship. Not only is this the most stable arrangement for your grandchildren (short of adoption), but if you apply for guardianship early enough, it can keep you out of the juvenile courts and prevent interference from child protective services. If your grandchildren's situation is not so severe or life threatening that you need to involve the police or child protective services, consider private guardianship (see "Guardianship," below).

▪ *Consider a power of attorney.* Power of attorney gives one person the legal right to make decisions for another. For instance, a single mother could give someone power of attorney to enroll a child in school or give emergency medical consent if she is out of town. In doing so, the mother doesn't give up any parental rights; she only allows another person to make certain decisions. Power of attorney can be a useful temporary solution when a parent is incarcerated and wants a relative to care for a child or when a parent travels extensively. Of course, a document like this is only useful if officials choose to accept it, and it can always be rescinded. If you are in a situation that does not require or allow for guardianship, at least ask the parents about power of attorney.

Court Placement and Foster Care

Foster care provides temporary substitute parenting to children whose parents can not or will not take care of them. It is part of an emergency response system that is designed to protect children who are suspected of being abused or neglected or who have been abandoned. Foster care usually starts with a call to a social worker, the police, or a child abuse hotline. The children are then taken into protective custody while the juvenile justice system decides whether or not to remove them from their parents and make them "dependents of the court."

Custody of your grandchild changes when she becomes a dependent of the court. The court retains legal custody of the child, but someone is awarded physical custody. That someone has traditionally been a foster parent. Foster parents are appointed to care for a child while the court conducts a series of hearings to determine if the allegations against the parents are true and, if so, how to protect the child. These hearings are generally called "dependency hearings."

Most people associate foster care with care by strangers. However, because of a shortage of foster homes and an explosion in the number of children needing court protection, many states have begun to rely increasingly on relatives. This makes court placement the most common *legal* arrangement for grandparents, although few grandparents are licensed foster parents.

With court placement, grandparents have a limited degree of custody. You have physical custody of the child (i.e., he lives with you) and limited authority to enroll him in school and seek medical attention, but the court and child welfare agency retain legal custody. Court placement gives you more legal protection than does an informal custody arrangement—and the possibility of higher government benefits—but you also have a kind of marriage to the juvenile justice system. You will be expected to comply with court visitation, to encourage "reunification" with the parents, and to submit your family to the scrutiny of the local child welfare agency. You exchange the possibility of parental interference for the certainty of interference by social workers, attorneys, and judges (and generally without any choice in the matter).

There are differences between court placement with a relative and foster care, mainly in terms of licensing requirements and government assistance. Foster parents must be trained and licensed to have children in their homes. They may be licensed only for a fixed number of children, for certain ages, and sometimes for one sex. They must also supply separate bedrooms for girls and boys and one bed per child. Many states also limit the number of children per room. Although relatives must also be approved by social services before a child can be placed with them, they don't usually have to go through the training and licensing process. Nor are housing guidelines so specific (in most states). Few grandparents could meet the strict criteria to become official foster parents.

The other difference between court placement with a relative and foster care is one of financial aid. Federal funds are available to support children who are in the custody of the state, and foster care benefits are significantly higher than welfare benefits. Some states also provide their own programs for children who don't qualify for federal foster care. Children placed with relatives are also entitled to government support, but relatives may have a harder time meeting federal foster care requirements and few states make state programs available to them. Families often have to rely on the smaller welfare benefits. (See Chapter 12 for more information on government aid.)

If you have a grandchild in the juvenile justice system, the individual laws of your state will determine if he is placed in your custody and under what conditions. The best thing you can do is educate yourself about the dependency process and try to comply with your state regulations. (See Chapter 11 for a discussion of child protective services and the dependency system.)

Guardianship

Outside of adoption, guardianship is the safest, most stable arrangement for a grandparent raising a grandchild. In fact, guardianship *is* custody, both physical and legal. It is the legal transfer of custody to someone other than a parent when one or both of the parents are dead, missing, or unfit. The first two categories are straightforward; "unfit" is a murkier concept. Nevertheless, unfit parents are becoming a common cause of guardianship actions. As attorney Teresa de la O told the Santa Rosa *Press Democrat*, "We've always done them [guardianships], but it used to be when one parent died and the other wasn't all that interested in having the child. Now we're doing it because neither parent is parenting."[8]

Guardianship does not terminate parental rights, but it does suspend them. With guardianship, you acquire rights and responsibilities that are similar, if not equal, to those of a parent. As attorney Harold LaFlamme puts it: "You step into the shoes of the parent. You don't have a pink slip, but something close."[9]

The advantage of guardianship is control. You decide where your grandchild lives (within the state). You have legal authority to enroll her in school, consent to medical treatment, and make many of the decisions a parent can make in terms of education, sports, health care, employment, and legal actions. You also have control over when and how your grandchild sees her parents, unless there is a court-ordered visitation schedule. The parent may retain some rights, similar to joint custody in a divorce settlement, but you have legal control. And you are not at the beck and call of the juvenile court system.

What you cannot do as a guardian is make decisions about the child's religion or move the child out of state without the court's permission. Although you are not entitled to any of the child's earnings or property, you also bear no financial responsibility for your grandchild. You are only responsible for the care and safety of the child and for any damage she does while you are guardian.

The disadvantages of applying for guardianship are the cost and the risk. Filing for private guardianship can mean high attorney fees and court costs, particularly if the parents or other relatives contest your petition. If guardianship comes through the juvenile court system, it can mean, for some families, a reduction in government foster care benefits, something many grandparents cannot afford to lose.

There are also emotional risks in filing for guardianship. Unless the parents have died or disappeared, you are petitioning to suspend parental rights. This requires proving that the parent is unfit and detrimental to the child. You will have to build a case against the parent that involves more than the separation anxiety your grandchild will suffer if he is removed from your home. You will have to show things like a history of irresponsibility, drug abuse, physical or sexual abuse, or a lack of residence, as well as the effect such factors will have on the child. You will also have to prove that it is in the child's best interests to be with you. You will not endear yourself to your adult child by painting these pictures and taking custody of the child. If you win, you guarantee some security for your grandchild. But, warns attorney LaFlamme, "If you lose, you could lose big: the money and the relationship with your child and grandchild."[10]

Even at its best, guardianship is never permanent. Under normal circumstances, it lasts until the child is 18,[11] marries, becomes emancipated (recognized as an adult), or is adopted. However, you can be removed as a guardian by the court at any time if it is proven that returning your grandchild to the parents or assigning another guardian is in the child's best interests. Only adoption offers airtight custody.

Filing for Guardianship

To file for private guardianship, you or your attorney must file several legal forms, often called a "guardianship petition," in whichever branch of your civil court handles guardianship (generally either probate, juvenile, or family law). You must also notify in writing all the child's maternal and paternal relatives, particularly the parents. These family members will be notified of all hearings and given an opportunity to object to your petition and to seek custody for themselves. You will also have to pay filing and investigation fees, the cost of which can vary.

If there is an emergency situation or you believe the child is at immediate risk and in need of protection, you can often ask the court to grant you "temporary guardianship"[12] until the hearing. This is one way to keep the children safe with you while you file for custody.

Once a hearing date is set, a state or county agency will conduct an investigation to decide if the guardianship is necessary. In most states the social service agency will also run a background check on you for any arrests or involvement with child protective services. The agency may also conduct an investigation of your home and may interview your grandchild if she is old enough. At the guardianship hearing, the judge will consider the petition, the social service investigator's report, and all the available testimony before making a final decision.

If there is no opposition to your petition from parents or other relatives, seeking guardianship can be a relatively simple procedure. If, however, the parents or other relatives contest your guardianship petition, they can hire their own attorneys and confront you in a full hearing. This is where the cost of court and attorney fees can start to climb.

Guardianship through Dependency

It is possible to obtain guardianship through the juvenile justice system but only at the final stages of the dependency process. If by the final hearing the judge decides that the child cannot safely return home, he or she will order adoption, guardianship, or long-term foster care as the best plan for the child. If guardianship is granted, the court may dismiss the child's dependency status. (For more on the dependency process, see Chapter 11. See also "Foster Care and Youakim" in Chapter 12.)

Standby and Short-Term Guardianship

A "standby guardianship" is a guardianship order issued with the parent's consent for some point in the future.[13] For instance, if a single mother has cancer, she can set up a standby guardianship that takes effect upon her death (as long as there is no other parent to object and the court doesn't find it harmful to the child). Short-term guardianship is just that: a legal custody arrangement for a limited period of time. Illinois just instituted the short-term guardianship in 1994. That state's "guardianship of limited duration" allows parents to appoint guardians for their child with a predetermined termination date.[14] This allows incarcerated parents to provide legal care for their children while they serve time and still regain custody upon their release.

If you are caring for a child whose parents are sick or in jail, find out if your state offers standby or short-term guardianship arrangements.

▪ WHAT YOU NEED TO KNOW

▪ *Sometimes court costs can be waived.* In some states you can apply for a waiver of court fees and costs if you can show financial hardship. The application is sometimes called a pauper's waiver or *in forma pauperis* application.[15] If you currently receive financial assistance for yourself (not your grandchild) in the form of disability or welfare benefits, food stamps, or any other form of general relief, you may qualify for this waiver.

▪ *You may be able to "do it yourself."* Some states make it possible to apply for guardianship without an attorney, particularly if the guardianship petition is uncontested. California grandparents can find guidance in *The Guardianship Book: How to Become a Child's Guardian in California* (Nolo Press)[16]; there may be manuals and booklets explaining the process in other states as well. If you don't need or cannot afford an attorney, find out if you can apply for guardianship without one. Contact your local Legal Aid office for information.

▪ *You must prove that it is harmful to the child to continue in the parent's custody.* Just because you are currently raising your grandchild is not enough reason for a judge to make you a guardian. Parents have a right to ask someone else to care for a child, particularly when they are in and out of the picture, without it being considered abandonment. If, on the other hand, the parent has disappeared for a significant amount of time, you may have a better chance for guardianship to be granted.

▪ *You must also show that the child is better off with you.* Be careful when you do this; reasons like better income can backfire. Says Pamela Mohr, attorney and executive director of the Alliance for Children's Rights, "It can work against you if it appears that you are wealthy and are trying to get the child for that reason. It makes the court protective of the parent. We don't want to take custody from poor people just because they are poor."[17] What kind of information is the court looking for? Information about the physical and emotional health of the child; how the child behaves after visits with the parent;

proof of your ability to provide a stable home environment if the parents cannot.

▪ *Parents will often be granted visitation rights.* A parent who doesn't have custody is entitled to reasonable visitation in a guardianship situation, unless the court decides that visitation poses a danger to the child's physical, mental, or emotional health. Even jailed parents may be granted visits if the court believes that they are in the best interests of the child. If either parent is granted visitation, be prepared to cooperate.

▪ *You can protect your grandchildren.* As a legal guardian you can determine where and when an unstable parent sees your grandchild. You can even get a restraining order, if necessary. But you must be able to show the court that the parent is a threat to you or to your grandchild's safety. Many grandparents won't get restraining orders against their adult children in fear of retaliation. It can also be difficult to call the police on your own son or daughter. But if you do have to call the police, a restraining order gives you more credibility.

▪ *Guardianship is always temporary.* Even if your grandchild has lived with you since birth, the court can revoke your guardianship status. Remember, the prevailing belief is that children belong with their parents. However, while parents can request the court to overturn a guardianship arrangement, they must prove that they can care for the child and that continued guardianship is no longer necessary. This is rarely accomplished when the problem is substance abuse.

Pam and Robert Marshall clearly understand this. They filed for custody of their granddaughter when the drug-addicted mother, Linda, was in jail (the father is unknown). "I know that guardianship can be overturned," says Pam, "but what it does is temporarily protect Megan. Linda would have to go into court and prove she has a home, a job, stability and could take care of her. As of yesterday, I doubt that."

▪ *Don't give up.* People will tell you many things. For instance, several attorneys told Pam Marshall that no court would allow her to take custody of a granddaughter. While it is possible that your state laws may prevent you from filing for guardianship, don't just take anyone's word for it. "No matter what anyone tells you, do it anyway," says one grandmother. "I was told I could not win. And you know what? I have three healthy, happy grandchildren."

Adoption

In many states you can adopt your own grandchildren under certain circumstances: for example, when the child is orphaned or legally abandoned, when the parents consent to the adoption, or when their parental rights are terminated by trial or the juvenile court system.

Adoption is the most secure custody arrangement available to nonparents. It permanently dissolves all legal ties between parent and child and creates a new parent–child relationship in the eyes of the law. In effect, you would no longer be grandparents to your grandchild but new parents, with all the rights and responsibilities of a biological parent. To quote one child welfare agency, "When you adopt a child, your legal relationship with that child is the same as with a child born to you."[18]

Adoption gives you full legal custody. It means the end of continual court appearances, and it means that the parent can never again contest or interfere. As an adoptive parent you can now put your grandchild on your health plan and allow her to inherit directly from you. You also acquire the full legal and financial responsibility for parenting the child. Unlike guardianship, adoption means that your relationship is permanent, extending past the child's 18th birthday, just as with your own children.

Adoption also means peace of mind, not only for you but for your grandchildren, who don't have to worry about ever being taken away again. Nancy Harper's granddaughter Marissa was thrilled when her grandmother adopted her. She thought it was wonderful that the judge said that she could stay with Grandma for the rest of her life and never leave. I heard about a little boy who took his stuffed bear to court with him. When the judge asked about it, he replied, "Well, he's always been at my Grandma's too, and he wants to know if he can be adopted, too, because he never wants to leave Grandma's house, either." Today, both boy and bear are legally adopted.

If adoption is such an airtight solution to the custody nightmares, you might ask, "why don't more grandparents pursue it?" There are several reasons.

■ *Grandparents don't easily give up on their adult children, and adoption means terminating the rights of the parent.* It can be a difficult emotional choice to make. On one hand, adopting a grandchild is a relief: It validates the fact that you are raising your grandchild and ends your dealings with social workers and the courts. On the other hand, it means admitting defeat where your adult child is concerned. Says attorney Robert Walmsley, "In terms of the grandparents, adoption is generally the last resort, when they see no hope of the adult child ever being responsible. Parenthood is precious. You hoped your child would shape up. By this point, you've lost all hope."[19]

▪ *Many grandparents believe that adoption is unnecessary because they and the children are already family.* They may also hesitate to adopt because the parents are still in the picture. The fact that the birth parents may continue to interact with the children can make grandparent adoption confusing and complicated. Because ties are not severed, children may be confused about whom to listen to and may be prevented from making a clean start with Grandma and Grandpa as a new family.

▪ *It is difficult to terminate a parent's rights.* Unless the parents consent to the adoption, have already lost custody, or are completely out of the picture, you may need to prove that your own child is unfit to raise his or her own children. This can involve a full trial with witnesses; everything about your family will be open to scrutiny.

▪ *Adoption is costly.* Not only do you have court costs, but unless your grandchildren are eligible for adoption assistance, you can also lose access to government aid. Many grandparents don't adopt their grandchildren because they live on a fixed income and can't afford to raise children without welfare benefits.

▪ *Your age can become a negative factor if the adoption is contested.* One New Hampshire couple had legal guardianship of their son's two children for two years before filing for adoption. Fourteen months into the trial, a young couple on the mother's side contested the adoption and won.

If you are considering adopting your grandchild, here are some things you might want to consider:

- You will be a full legal parent again. Are you ready for that?
- Will the parents continue to interact with the child? How will you handle that?
- Does the child have a relationship with the parents? How will adoption affect that relationship?
- How is your health? Do you have the stamina and good health to commit to raising another set of children?

- What is your financial situation? If you are getting government aid, can you afford to give it up? Are you eligible for Adoption Assistance (see Chapter 12)?

If you decide to go ahead with the adoption, consult a good adoption attorney—as well as a therapist about the impact this move could have on your grandchild and your family. If the child is old enough, listen closely to what he or she has to say about it. Some children are eager to cut their ties to their parents, others will object.

VISITATION

Legal visitation is not a form of custody, but it is an important issue when the custody of a child changes. In a divorce, for instance, the mother may get legal custody and the father may receive visitation privileges. The grandparents can sometimes be left out in the cold. However, divorce is not the only situation in which grandparents are prevented from seeing their grandchildren. Grandparents may also be denied visitation in the following circumstances:

- A daughter dies and the husband remarries.
- An unmarried son fathers a child and the mother moves away.
- A stepparent adopts the grandchildren.
- A grandchild is placed in foster care.
- A married daughter simply refuses to let her parents see their grandchildren.

Even grandparents who have raised a child for years can lose total access to that child if the parents reappear or regain custody. One Ohio grandmother provided day care for her married daughter for 50 hours a week for four years; after a family argument, the parents refused her even occasional visitation. In situations like these, many grandparents turn to the law for help.

Grandparent Visitation and State Laws

Nearly every state in the United States has some kind of grandparent visitation statute, although they are barely 30 years old and narrow in scope.[20] These statutes do not give grandparents a legal right to visit a grandchild but a right to *petition* for visitation. The court reserves the right to refuse any petition based on the merits of the case. Each statute defines who may petition for visitation, when, and under what circumstances. Some states also outline what standard the court should apply in awarding visitation, usually "the best interests of the child."

▪ *Who may petition.* While most states only allow grandparents to petition for visitation, a number of states extend the privilege to great-grandparents, siblings, and other relatives.

▪ *When you may petition.* The majority of states limit the right to petition to specific circumstances, such as the divorce or death of a parent. However, some states include additional circumstances, such as incarceration of the parent; abuse, neglect, or abandonment of the child; juvenile delinquency; and when custody has been given to a third party or when the child has been placed in foster care. Others even allow grandparents to seek visitation when the parents are still married or when the parents are unmarried. Although adoption usually cuts all ties between a child and his or her biological family, a few states allow grandparents to petition for visitation in instances when a grandchild has been adopted by a stepparent or other relative.[21]

Visitation statutes, however, are relatively new in U.S. law. Many have not yet been tested at the court level and have no case law to back them up. Even those that have been upheld by the courts have little in the way of legislation or procedures to enforce them, and because there is no uniformity from state to state, a parent who really wants to prevent visitation can always move.

Visitation in Dependency

If a child is removed from the parents by child protective services and is not placed with you, the court may consider whether it is in his best interests to have visits with you. Many factors can influence this decision, including your prior relationship with the child and whether such visitation might interfere with parental reunification.

If the parents' rights are terminated by the court, your relationship with your grandchild could terminate as well. Some states do allow grandparents to petition for visitation when a child is adopted by a stepparent or relative but not when the adoptive parents are unrelated.

▪ HOW TO COPE

▪ *Know the law.* Visitation laws vary. Find out the parameters of your own state's visitation laws and proceed accordingly.

▪ *Consider alternatives to legal action.* Litigation is not only expensive but also time-consuming, and it can permanently damage already fragile family relationships. Once a lawsuit starts, people cling to their own side of the story and stop listening. Animosity grows. The children are the ones who get caught in the cross fire. Furthermore, while people's feelings constantly change and evolve, court decisions are fixed and inflexible. Is there anything you can do to keep your family out of the courtroom? Would family counseling address the parent's unwillingness to allow visitation? Is mediation a possibility? Some states have informal dispute resolution or mediation services to help settle visitation problems. If you must battle in court to see your grandchild, it can certainly be worth the fight, but first try to seek other alternatives.

▪ *Take heart.* Although the law once gave complete weight to the rights of the parent, public opinion concerning the rights and well-being of the child has influenced the courts. Increasingly, the courts are recognizing that a child's well-being involves a stable relationship with grandparents. As one New Jersey Supreme Court jurist put it, "It is a biological fact that grandparents are bound to their grandchildren by the unbreakable link of heredity. Visits with a grandparent are often a precious part of a child's experience."[22]

WHEN YOU NEED AN ATTORNEY

At some point in this second parenthood you may need to consult an attorney. Perhaps your grandchild has ended up as a dependent of the court and you risk losing her to the system. Perhaps you are trying for guardianship. Maybe you don't have your grandchild, but you are petitioning for visitation rights. Each of these can be an overwhelming legal battle, and you may want an expert on your side. Even if you are settled in a comfortable custody situation, there are other wars to fight on behalf of your grandchild—with various agencies for proper government aid; with your school district for proper educational services; even with hospitals and Medicaid for medical coverage. Although you are your grandchild's best advocate, sometimes even the sharpest advocate needs help.

Do You Need Legal Counsel?

Whether or not you need an attorney depends on what it is you are trying to accomplish. If everything is going smoothly or you are filing an uncontested visitation and guardianship agreement, you may not need an attorney. Much will depend on the laws of your state.

On the other hand, you do want to hire an attorney whenever the parent or parents hire one first; it keeps the playing field level. You may also need an attorney if you are contesting a judicial proceeding, petitioning to become part of a proceeding, filing a contested visitation or guardianship petition, adopting a child, or appealing an administrative decision.

If you have a question you can't answer, you may need to consult with an attorney, but you may not need to hire one to represent you. Consultation fees vary. Each state has its own laws about when you can and cannot legally represent yourself, but one thing is certain: If you feel you need an attorney, you should consider hiring one.

What to Look For

Attorneys, like doctors, have different specialties. This is true even within the field of family law. If you petition for guardianship, you don't want an attorney who specializes in divorce or dependency. And if a dependency hearing is imminent, you need an attorney who really knows the juvenile justice system. "People buy a car and read *Consumer Reports* and investigate," says attorney Michael Salazar. "But when it comes to picking a lawyer, they assume the first lawyer they find will be an expert. This is an exact specialty, like brain surgery."[23] In other words, know what you're looking for, and do your research.

When you look for legal counsel, you also want to make sure your case is not the first grandparent case your attorney has ever handled. Although this is, indeed, a new area of law, you don't want to be someone's maiden voyage if you can help it. This is where knowledge is power. Learn the terms. Then make sure your attorney knows them. Does he understand the ins and outs of the dependency process? Can he discuss changes in visitation law? If not, find someone who can.

It is just as important to make sure your attorney believes in your case. When a South Carolina couple wanted to mount a legal battle for their grandson, they were discouraged by an attorney who told them, "He's got parents."[24] This is not an attorney you want working for you.

Where to Look

Where you look for an attorney or an advocate depends on your resources and circumstances. Attorneys charge by the hour, and their rates vary according to your location, the size of their firm, and the difficulty of the case. Your total cost will also depend on what needs to be accomplished; filing a document will cost considerably less than a protracted fight in court. One grandmother's attorney told her that her custody battle with the child's mother would cost her "a room addition and a trip to Europe" before they were finished, and he wasn't far off. On the other hand, some cases can be simple and straightforward.

Your best source for legal referrals are other grandparents and grandparent support groups. Which attorneys have other people worked with? What were their experiences? They know which ones are effective and which ones are not. Also, if you are involved in a dependency case, you might consider asking the court clerks which lawyers they recommend. "Everyone knows who they'd hire if they were in trouble, and the ones they'd stay away from," says attorney Michael Salazar.[25]

If you are on a fixed income, you will have a smaller pool to choose from, but you still have options. Ask your state or local bar association if any family law attorneys work "pro bono" (i.e., donate legal assistance) or at reduced rates. Contact your local Legal Aid society or legal services office to find out about free or low-cost representation for people who are income eligible. A law school or law clinic might even provide voluntary services to people on fixed or limited incomes. These organizations may be shy about helping you because of the newness of grandparent litigation and their own inexperience with the issues, but don't be afraid to ask. Every day and with every case, grandparent issues lose their novelty, and organizations like Legal Aid are sure to recognize the growing need for legal assistance.

Court-Appointed Attorneys

Many states offer court-appointed attorneys to key parties in a dependency case who cannot afford their own attorneys, namely, parents who have been accused of abusing or neglecting their children and, sometimes, the children themselves. A court-appointed attorney has the same obligations as a private attorney in terms of representing her clients in court. Occasionally, a grandparent or relative will be eligible for a court-appointed attorney. Some states allow relatives and foster parents who have acted as day-to-day parents in a child's life to petition for "de facto parent"[26] status and become a party in a case, which gives them the right to legal representation. If these de facto parents cannot afford an attorney, the court may be able to appoint one for them.

While a court-appointed attorney can be a financial help, this method of acquiring legal counsel can be a game of Russian roulette in terms of an attorney's sensitivity. You could get a compassionate, caring individual who truly supports your case or one of those who are just doing their job. One grandmother's court-appointed attorney, speaking to me on behalf of her client, told me she was "dumb as dirt" and "too emotional." The risk is even greater when the only attorney in the picture is a court-appointed attorney for the child. In this case, he is only bound to represent the child. Whether or not your view is ever heard will depend on the attorney and how sympathetic that individual is to grandparents.

If your court-appointed attorney is wonderful, treasure her. Unfortunately, there isn't much you can do if you're unhappy with your attorney. You can request a replacement, but you may not get one.

▪ HOW TO COPE

▪ *Be persistent.* If your attorney doesn't return your calls in a timely fashion, keep calling back. Attorneys have busy schedules and busy office staffs; sometimes messages fall through the cracks.

▪ *Tell your attorney the whole truth.* Tell the negative as well as the positive. Don't hide anything. Withholding information because you fear it could hurt your case can do more damage than telling the truth. If you have something in your past that could cause trouble—for instance, a jail record from your youth—let your attorney know. He can address the problem in a way that could minimize damage to your case. If you don't tell him, and the other side finds out, they could have a field day in court.

"Every lawyer assumes his client has not told him all the things that he would like to know," says attorney Charles Ollinger. "Sometimes it's intentional. Sometimes it doesn't occur to a client to mention [something]. It is surprising how important those [facts] can be upon occasion."[27]

CHAPTER 11

Child Protection and the Dependency System

> You have to have an understanding of what the dependency law is, for a grandparent, to understand what kind of Pandora's box you are opening when you make that one call to CPS [Child Protective Services].
> —*Ted Youmans, attorney*[1]

Claire and Evan Powers basically raised their granddaughter, Sarah, until she was 10 years old. Sarah had arrived in the world with the deck stacked against her: a father who drank, a mother on drugs, and an abusive relationship between the two. Claire and Evan, her father's parents, were her ace in the hole; they often let her mother stay the night or agreed to keep the baby with them when violence broke out at home. Almost from the beginning, Sarah was in and out of Grandma's house.

Then, when Sarah was 18 months old, her parents split up. Dad wanted the baby off the streets, so Mom and Sarah moved in with Evan and Claire. In a few months Mom disappeared without warning, and with Sarah. When the father found her in a crack house six months later, he sued for custody. One day while the case was still pending, Mom showed up with Sarah. "I can't take care of her anymore; I'll be back in three months," she told Claire, and took off. Dad got custody of two-year-old Sarah, but Grandma and Grandpa got the bulk of the responsibility. For the next four years they bought her clothes, took her to the day-care center, and baby-sat, sometimes for a week at a time. Sarah was spending more and more time at Grandma's house, and eventually father and daughter moved in with Evan and Claire.

By this time, however, Dad was also using drugs and was increasingly abusive to his parents and his daughter. He moved into a motel near a crack house. One day he decided he didn't want his parents to have Sarah; he packed her up and took her down to the crack house with him. Claire called the sheriff. She had called child abuse hotlines three times before because of her son's drug use and child abuse, but each time she was told there was not enough evidence. This time there was. Sarah's father was arrested at the crack house; Sarah was taken into protective custody, then placed back with Claire. Finally, Claire thought, her problems were over. Little did she know they were just beginning.

When Claire called the sheriff, she started the wheels of justice turning. The wheels of justice, she discovered, sometimes run over the very people they are meant to help. The social services agency not only started dependency court proceedings against the father but went out looking for Mom, who had not been seen in several years.

Sarah's mother had been a heavy drug user for most of the eight years of Sarah's life. She knew where her daughter was, but she never had contact with her. She didn't send her letters, and she didn't offer support. She had no parental relationship with the child, who barely knew her. She was living on the streets when they found her. Still, the system offered her a free lawyer, reunification services, a drug rehabilitation program, and, eventually, Sarah. Even though she had essentially abandoned the child. Even though she had been investigated for child abuse three times before Sarah was six months old. Even though the child told everyone—the social worker, the judge, the attorney, her grandparents and her mother—that she didn't want to go with her mother, that the only home she had was with Grandma and Grandpa. "Sarah jumped up on my lap in court and hugged me; I was crying," Claire recalls. "She thought she was going home with me because she had told the judge that she wanted to."

Today Sarah is 12 years old. She has lost weight, has trouble sleeping, and is developing behavioral problems. Claire and Evan can only see her for one weekend each month, and achieving that right cost them $35,000 in legal fees. The mother doesn't make it easy, either: Visits are never hassle free, and she sends Sarah to her grandparents for three days with only the clothes on her back. "She would like people to believe she's clean, but I don't think she is," says Claire. "Even the judge said, at the time, that the mother has unresolved drug problems and the boyfriend is an alcoholic, but he had to protect the mother's visitation rights. These were visitation rights she'd had for years and never used."

Claire and Evan Powers lost their granddaughter by calling a system they thought would help them. Claire says that call was "the biggest mistake ever." The system protects the parents. It gives them attorneys and it gives them services. "They follow them around with a pillow so if they fall down they don't get bruised," she says bitterly.

"The system." Grandparents shudder when they talk about it. Two words that seem to stand for everything impersonal, overbearing, and bureaucratic in government. Power gone out of control. When grandparents talk about "the system," they mean the dependency system, the combination of child protection agencies and juvenile court proceedings that are designed to protect and aid children in crisis.

Many grandparents have never dealt with the system before now, having raised their own children without contact with courts and social workers. Even those who are familiar with the juvenile courts find that involvement as a grandparent is completely different from involvement as a parent. In any case, the dependency process can be an overwhelming and frustrating experience. Every grandparent needs to know about this process—not only to protect themselves if they find themselves in the system but to learn when and how to avoid it. And why.

WHAT IS THE DEPENDENCY SYSTEM?

The dependency system is part of the government's emergency response to protect minor children who are suspected of being abused, neglected, or abandoned. Every state has at least one part of its child welfare agency that is dedicated to investigating reports of children in crisis—often called child protective services (CPS)—and at least one court, typically, the juvenile court, responsible for deciding these cases.

The dependency process is a series of hearings in which a judge decides whether or not allegations against the parents* are true and,

---

* For simplicity, we are using the plural "parents" throughout this discussion. It is understood that in many cases only one parent may be involved.

if so, how to protect the child while the parents try to solve their problems. Among the issues considered in the various dependency hearings are the following:

- Whether the child should be removed from the home
- Where the child should be placed during the dependency process
- What measures, such as drug rehabilitation and counseling, the parents must take to regain custody of the child
- What the court can do to help the parents reunite with the child (for example, devise a visitation schedule or order parenting classes)
- What services, such as counseling, the court can recommend for the child
- How the family is progressing
- If and when the child can safely return home
- What permanent custody arrangement can be made if the child cannot return home (permanent plans are generally a choice of adoption, guardianship, or long-term foster care)

During the course of these hearings the child is considered a "dependent of the court" (thus the term "dependency hearings"). This means that legal custody of the child transfers from the parents to the state (whereas physical custody will be awarded to someone who can care for the child). The dependency system is, for many children, the entrance door into foster care, although a number of states give preference to placing children with relatives.

Dependency hearings are the most powerful court proceedings connected with a child. Once CPS intervenes and juvenile court takes jurisdiction, you and your grandchild are locked into the system for a defined period of time. Decisions are taken out of the hands of your family and placed in the hands of the court; parents and grandparents lose control of the situation. In most states the dependency system has exclusive jurisdiction; it overrules all other courts, including family law and guardianship.[2] This means that while the case is active in the dependency process, no other court can make decisions about the child. In other words, once your grandchild goes into the system, you are married to the courts for as long as the process lasts. For a grandparent, this can pose serious problems:

- *Dependency is a nightmare of bureaucracy.* Everyone in the system seems to work against each other. Caseloads are high. Communication within the system is poor. Sometimes critical information never reaches the attending judge. One child welfare agency director describes dependency as "a mass custody suit where six to eight different interests are represented." Often, the ones who lose are the children.

▪ *The dependency process is a mystery because it is confidential.* Most cases are closed except to the parties involved—generally, the child, the parents, and the child welfare department. This means that the public and the press cannot come into these courtrooms the way they may come into criminal and civil courts. You may not be allowed to speak on behalf of your grandchildren, even if you are raising them, unless you have "standing" (see "How to Cope," below).

▪ *Dependency is relentless.* Although there are state and federal time lines for when certain hearings must take place, attorneys often waive these deadlines, and the process can drag on—sometimes for years.

▪ *Dependency splinters families.* When you are in the dependency process, you are at the mercy of strangers. I have seen social workers decide that Grandma is too old, too overbearing, or too possessive to have a child (or, in one case, not "grieving properly"). They pull children out of the grandparents' home and place them in foster care or a group home; the grandparents might not even get visitation rights. If this happens and if the parents' rights are terminated, your role as grandparent will also end.

▪ *Dependency favors parents.* The dependency system does not worry about grandparents. When social workers and judges talk about keeping families together, they mean biological parents and children. Grandparents don't count as "legal" family and have little credibility in court. "In court, you are not seen as reliable people speaking for the child; you are looked upon as meddlers," says attorney Ted Youmans. "It's terrifying to get involved with the system and realize someone else has control over a member of your family."[3]

The catchphrase in the dependency system is "family reunification." This means that, except in very limited circumstances, the social service agency will work to enable parents to regain custody of their children. Toward that end, the system will offer parents all kinds of services to help them correct the problems that led to their losing custody and to help them "reunify" with their children. The presumption is that children belong with their parents and parents should have every opportunity to raise their own children. Says Judge Lawrence L. Koontz, Jr., of Virginia, "The goal of the court is to restore custody to one of the natural parents whenever possible."[4]

Meanwhile, you, as a relative caregiver, must encourage this parent–child relationship if the child is to be placed with you. The court will place a child with strangers rather than let family members interfere with reunification. This can be devastating, particularly if you are prevented from seeing or contacting your grandchild. Grandparents repeatedly get lost and overwhelmed in the maze of steps and hearings that make up the dependency process. Here, as everywhere, knowledge is your best defense.

DEPENDENCY: STEP BY STEP

Dependency law is extensive and complex. This discussion is only a general blueprint of the process; it is designed as a tool to help you ask questions about the laws and regulations in your own state. Although each stage of the dependency process has various possible outcomes, each stage explained below assumes, for simplicity's sake, that the child has been removed from the home and placed with relatives. The schedule used in this discussion reflects Los Angeles County procedures. Your own state laws may outline more steps, different names, and a different time line.

The Call

A parent is arrested or injured, and no one is around to take the children. A child is left alone in an apartment for hours. A teacher suspects a student is being abused at home. The dependency process starts with a call to child protective services about a child who is suspected of being abandoned, neglected, or abused. CPS then sends out an emergency response social worker to investigate the situation.

Anyone can call CPS about a child at risk, including clergy, neighbors, and family members. Some states also have a list of "mandated reporters," that is, individuals who are required by law to report any suspicion of child abuse or neglect (e.g., teachers, doctors, therapists, and child care providers.) When the investigation takes place depends on the nature of the allegation. A call about suspected abuse generally receives more immediate attention than a call about neglect. Even if the caller can provide an address but no name, CPS must respond.

Depending on what the social worker finds, one of several things can happen:

- The case can be dismissed for lack of evidence.
- The parents may agree to seek counseling, rehabilitation, or other services to correct the problem, and the child remains in the home. The court may or may not get involved.
- The child may be considered to be "at risk" and removed from parental custody.

Of course, what social workers actually find during an investigation often depends on when they visit and how thorough they are. A worker who makes an immediate unannounced visit, for instance, will often see a different picture than one who makes an appointment. Even a day's notice can give neglectful parents time to clean the house, stock the refrigerator, and generally make a better appearance.

The Pickup

If a social worker (or police officer) finds enough evidence to indicate that a child is in danger of abuse or neglect at home, the child will be taken into protective custody. Some states may release a child into the care of a relative if one shows up with proof of relationship and a clean background check. At this point the case can either be dismissed or referred to the juvenile court through a "petition of dependency" (see below). However, if no one comes to take the child or if for some reason CPS won't release him, the social worker must refer the case to the juvenile court for a hearing. During this time the child could be inaccessible to the family.

What You Need to Know

Keep track of your grandchildren. If you know they have been picked up by CPS, be persistent in locating them. Be sure to take birth certificates or something that proves your relationship to the children, especially if their last name is different from yours. Your actions may not prevent the dependency process from kicking into gear, but if CPS will release the children to you, it may make it easier for you to get placement down the line. At the very least, let the social worker know you are interested in placement or future visitation.

The Petition

A petition of dependency is the legal document that tells a judge why the social worker thinks the court should intervene to protect a child. In essence, it is the state's formal allegation against the parents for the abuse and neglect of a minor, and it formally requests that the child be made a dependent of the court. The petition must be filed within *48 court hours* (i.e., two working days) after the child is taken into protective custody.[5] It includes whatever facts the child welfare agency believes will support its claims and identifies the sections of the law under which the parents are accused; these accusations are important because they determine which programs the parents will have to complete in order to regain custody of the child. For instance, if the petition claims the child has been physically abused but there are no allegations of drug use, the court cannot send the parents to drug treatment.

The Detention Hearing

The detection hearing (sometimes known as "arraignment and detection," "shelter care hearing," or "temporary custody hearing") is the first judicial proceeding in a dependency case, the hearing that sets the case in motion. It is a quick hearing, without much investigation beforehand and with just a brief report from the emergency response worker.

At the detention hearing the parents are formally informed of the reason the child was taken into temporary custody and the allegations against them. This is also the stage where parents are informed of their right to an attorney. If they cannot afford one, some states will appoint one free of charge. Some states also appoint an attorney for the child; others use the same attorney who represents the child welfare agency (often called the Department of Social Services, or DSS).

Two issues are decided at the detention hearing stage: how the parents will respond to the allegations and whether there is enough evidence to detain the child in temporary custody until the court determines whether the allegations in the petition are true. If the parents do not dispute the charges, the case will go on to a disposition hearing. If the parents deny the charges, the case will move on to mediation or trial. The judge can also schedule another hearing to provide more information.

Courts are typically reluctant to take children from their parents, and this includes the child who has been taken into protective custody. If the judge can safely release a child to the parents, with DSS supervision, he or she usually will. However, if the child cannot be returned to the parents, she may be placed in a temporary foster home or with a relative until the case is resolved. It is also possible that the case could be dismissed at this point, with or without continued supervision by social services.

What You Need to Know

The detention hearing is a critical hearing. If you are aware of it, try to show up. You probably won't be able to attend—these hearings are confidential—but you can let the court officers, social workers, or child's attorney know, for the record, that you are a grandparent and want to be a resource. Many state laws give preference to placing children with relatives, but they have to know you exist. Social services will run a background and criminal check on you before you can take your grandchild home.

If the court won't consider you for placement, you might be able to request visitation while your grandchild is in the care of another relative or in foster care. The best-case scenario is that the child is placed with you. At worst, the child is taken from the parents and placed in a foster home and you don't find out about it for months. This is particularly common when grandparents live in another state.

Mediation and/or Trial

The decision-making phase of the dependency process involves mediation and/or trial. This is the stage where the court decides whether or not the allegations against the parents are true and, if so, whether or not the state will assume legal custody of the child. These determinations are generally made in a "jurisdictional hearing" (or trial), but some states try to avoid the need for a trial by settling the case through mediation.

Mediation Stage

Some states insert a mediation stage (sometimes called a "pretrial hearing" or a "pretrial resolution conference") between the detention and jurisdictional hearings. This is the state's attempt to settle a case without going to trial. Sometimes the allegations in the petition can be proven untrue and the case is dismissed. Sometimes a parent is willing to admit to the charges in the petition, or the petition can be amended to reflect charges a parent *will* admit to. For instance, Dad may have earlier denied the allegations of drug abuse but by the mediation stage may admit to occasional cocaine use. If a settlement is reached, the case could go directly to a "disposition hearing" (see below), sometimes even the same day. If, however, the parents continue to deny all allegations, the case goes to a jurisdictional hearing, or trial.

Trial Stage

If a settlement is not reached through mediation or if a state does not provide mediation services, the case goes into the trial phase of the dependency process. (This trial is also known as the adjudication or jurisdictional hearing.) DSS presents evidence that the child has been abused or neglected. The attorney for the parents questions the evidence and presents counterevidence. Witnesses may be called. Finally, the judge decides if the charges in the petition against the parents are true, which charges are true, and whether or not to make the child a dependent of the court. If the court finds the petition is not true, the case is dismissed and the child returned to the home. If the court finds the petition is true, the case is set for a disposition hearing.

What You Need to Know

It is important to understand which charges are proven or admitted at the trial stage; they will be important at the disposition hearing, when the court decides what plan the parents must follow to regain custody of the child. For instance, if a petition claims a parent has a drug problem and is physically abusive but the judge doesn't see enough evidence to prove drug abuse, the case plan cannot include drug rehabilitation services. However, if additional proof appears later on, DSS can often make new allegations or amend the petition, so make your grandchild's social worker aware of what you know— and can prove—as the case goes along.

The Disposition Hearing

If the allegations against the parents are judged to be true, the case goes to a disposition hearing. This is where the court decides what to do to both protect the child and help the parents regain custody. At or before the disposition hearing the child's social worker submits a report on the status of the case and a case plan recommending where the child should live, how often the parents should visit or call, and what services should be offered to the children and to the parents to improve conditions in the home and facilitate the return of the child to the parents.

The judge considers the social worker's report and recommendations, as well as evidence and arguments from other parties, before making a decision on the case. Final court orders typically include a "reunification plan," which stipulates what conditions the parents must fulfill in order to regain custody of the child, a visitation schedule, and a decision on placement for the child. The placement plan occasionally sends the child home with a parent under DSS supervision; more often, the child is placed in the home of a relative, a foster home, or a group home.

Periodic Reviews

Once the child has been placed with a relative or foster parents and reunification services have been offered to the parents, there will be periodic hearings (also known as "administrative case reviews," "judicial reviews," and "dependency status reviews") to review the family's progress. These reviews are conducted every six months by either the court or the child welfare agency and consider both the case and the case plan. The following questions are addressed: Is the case plan being followed? How are the parents progressing? Does the child need additional services? When might the child return to parental custody? If by the second review it seems unlikely that the child will return home, a permanent plan may be established. If the parents are doing well but are not quite ready to resume custody, the court can grant a six-month extension before deciding on the permanent plan.

What You Need to Know

Although relative caregivers may be entitled to receive notification of each review hearing in advance, they are rarely notified in time, if at all. Since you know these reviews are every six months, try to keep track of when they are scheduled. Let the judge, the child's lawyer, and the social worker know that you want to be informed of these hearings, and try to attend. Be prepared to talk about how you are complying with the reunification plan if you are asked and to provide comments and observations about the child's reactions to parental visits. This is another place careful documentation can be helpful. Also, keep records of all legal documents, bills, correspondence, and contacts with the lawyer, the social worker, the court, and the parents. If you write letters to the court, copy them to all the attorneys involved to make sure everyone reads them.

Permanency Planning Hearing

Federal law requires that a permanent plan for each child who enters the dependency system be established no later than 18 months from the date of the original placement.[6] At this point the child must either be safely returned to the parents or assigned to a permanent plan by the court. In either case, reunification services end. If a child cannot be returned home, the court has three options, in order of preference: adoption, guardianship, and long-term foster care. Adoption has the highest priority because it is the most permanent solution. Guardianship only lasts until the child is 18 years old, and it can be terminated before then. Long-term foster care is the least stable option.

What You Need to Know

Some social workers may try to pressure you into adopting your grandchild. Not only is it a more permanent plan for the child, but because it may end government benefits, it is less costly to the system. They are not supposed to pressure you. Although the courts do look at adoption as a first choice, there are reasons grandparents may not want to adopt, or even seek guardianship, of a grandchild: They may not be ready to give up on their adult children. They may be under financial stress and need the government aid. They may feel that their age or medical condition might rule out adoption.

"The truth is that the court looks at the relative caretaker very differently than they look at a nonrelated caretaker," says attorney Pamela Mohr. "They realize there is a familial obligation. Even if the kid is not legally your kid, the kid is your grandkid and will be your grandkid for the rest of your life. They aren't worried about your just abandoning the child."[7] (See "Adoption" in Chapter 10 and "Adoption Assistance Program" in Chapter 12.)

▪ HOW TO COPE

▪ *Find out about relative placement.* Federal law encourages state agencies to place children in the "least restrictive" environment.[8] This is often interpreted to mean placing children with family, when possible. Moreover, because of the shrinking number of available foster homes and the increasing number of children needing care, many states now have formal regulations and guidelines that give preference to placing children with relatives—often grandparents—before nonrelatives. If your grandchild is in the system—or runs a risk of ending up in the system—find out your state's policy on relative placement.

Of course, a state's preference for placing children with relatives doesn't guarantee that placement. The court must first evaluate your ability to provide a secure and stable home for the child. It will also consider your willingness to support visitation and reunification with the parent and whether or not you have a criminal record.

If your state does not support relative placement or if the child is not placed with you, you can still try to get visitation privileges. Stay as connected with your grandchild as you can, and let the social workers know if you are interested in permanent placement if the parent and child cannot reunify.

▪ *Start early!* It is critical that you express your concern for your grandchild as early in the dependency process as possible, especially if you want the child placed with you. Although many states require DSS to identify family resources, this is not always fully accomplished. There may not be enough time to look for family. Parents may be uncooperative about supplying names and phone numbers. Some social workers may simply neglect to interview relatives. Unfortunately, if too much time passes, the court may rule out relative placement altogether; the child may have bonded with foster parents, who may be considering adoption, and the court may be unwilling to disrupt the situation. "It's really a heartrending situation," says attorney Pamela Mohr. "There's no answer for those cases and, unfortunately, they're fairly common."[9] If you cannot locate your grandchild but suspect that she is in the system, contact child welfare in the child's last known location and let them know that you are a resource.

Even if you can't get placement early on, you can ask for visitation. This at least would allow you to continue your involvement in your grandchild's life, a fact that could be important if you later seek placement or custody. In fact, don't hesitate to let the social worker and the court know if you are willing to take your grandchild on a permanent basis in the event that the parents cannot fulfill the reunification requirements. The sooner you express your interest, the more likelihood you have of being considered.

▪ *Attend hearings!* Once your grandchild is in the system, attend every hearing that you can. You may not be permitted into the courtroom, but let the bailiff or the court clerk know, for the record, that you are there, that you are a grandparent, and that you are interested in placement or visitation. The fact that there exists a real person who is willing to take a child can sometimes affect a judge's decision. You can also write a letter to the judge. If you do, send copies to all the attorneys involved and keep it simple.

▪ *Ask about standing.* "Standing" is the right to participate in a case as a party, which means you are entitled to receive notice of hearings, to be represented by an attorney, and to present evidence. Although rules of the court often change from county to county in terms of who may speak in court, when they may do so, and under what circumstances, the parties who have standing in a dependency case are generally the parents, the child, and the child welfare agency. Grandparents and other relatives typically do not have standing in a dependency case; they may not even be permitted in the courtroom. However, some states will allow a person who has raised and provided for a child for some time to qualify as a *de facto* parent, that is, a parent "in actuality" or a substitute parent.[10] This person, whether related to the child or not, may be entitled to standing and in some cases to a court-appointed attorney. However, you may have to hire a private attorney in order to prove de facto parent status.

Some states allow relatives limited participation in a dependency case without full standing.[11] Judges also have the authority to let you in the courtroom if they want to hear what you have to say. Keep asking questions until you know exactly what kind of involvement you are entitled to in your court system.

▪ *Behave yourself in court.* Grandparents have an image problem in court. In their fury to protect their grandchildren (and their frustration with the system) they often argue with court clerks, attorneys, and even judges attempting to clarify the danger of the situation and the need to move quickly. Despite their best intentions this approach often backfires, and the grandparents become known as rabble-rousers and troublemakers. Social workers may forget to return their phone calls, court clerks may claim to have misplaced documents, and the court may turn a deaf ear to their concerns.[12] You will have more success if you follow two rules:

1. Be gracious with court officials. Remember that you are asking for help when you deal with the court system; you don't score points by making demands. "Clerks are in charge of what happens to papers," notes attorney Charles Ollinger. "The judge is in charge of what happens in the courtroom. When you go in there, you're playing in their ballpark, by their rules."[13]

2. Be polite in court. Don't interrupt or blurt out comments. Try to stay calm; avoid arguing with the parents in front of the judge. Cooperate with your attorney, if you have one. Above all, don't argue with the judge. (For more on court behavior see "A Word About Judges," below.)

▪ *Support reunification.* If you wish to have your grandchild placed with you, you have to not only keep your feelings about the parents private but actively work toward reuniting the parents with the child—even if you've seen them abuse your grandchild and even if you think reunification is the most horrible thing that could happen to your grandchild. If you cannot support reunification, the court may not place the child with you. It may not be able to. And if you speak or act against the parents while the child is living with you, social services can remove him. Of course, that doesn't mean you must let a parent see a child when he or she shows up intoxicated on your doorstep, but it does mean you must do everything else to actively encourage reunification.

▪ *Be prepared for delays.* From the moment the child is removed, a clock starts ticking. According to federal law, a permanent plan must be established for a child no later than 18 months from the date of the original placement. However, it rarely happens that way. Marjorie Brown's granddaughter was six months old when she was placed with Marjorie and was three by the time a permanent plan was established. Sue Ellen Rice's grandson entered the system three years ago; he and his family have been in permanency planning hearings for almost a year now, as his mother continues to fight for custody.

Various factors contribute to these delays. Rising caseloads make scheduling difficult at every stage. Hearings may be continued over several dates to allow for further investigation or psychological evaluations. Attorneys may waive the time line on a client's case. Sympathetic judges may refrain from enforcing the time line, thus giving parents an additional chance to complete their requirements and prove themselves. There may also be discrepancies in when the court starts the clock. The phrase *original placement* leaves room for interpretation. According to attorney Michael Salazar, some cases can be in the system for two years without even going to trial.[14]

There may also be a conflict in the law itself, says attorney Pamela Mohr. Although federal law sets an 18-month time line on dependency cases, some states require that parents be offered at least 12 months of family reunification services. If those services only start at Month 16, there is a problem. Mohr encourages relatives to make sure services are really offered to parents from the beginning. "Even if the parents are hopeless," says Mohr, "if you really offer 12 months of reunification, the court will have less qualms about [letting you take the kids]."[15] It is difficult to really pressure the court in this instance. At least make sure your attorney really knows how to maneuver in the dependency system, and then find a support group where you can vent your frustrations with other grandparents.

HOTLINES ARE NOT ALWAYS HELP LINES

Claire Powers called a hotline to help her granddaughter; in the end she lost her. The system went out, found Mom, and pulled her back into the picture. And Mom came running. To quote one family law judge, "The most disinterested parent in the world becomes the most interested when someone tries to interfere with their God-given, constitutionally protected right to parent."

But this is not the only reason to avoid hotlines. If you call a child abuse hotline on your adult child and he or she finds out, you can bury yourself in the system. If your grandchild is removed from a parent, he or she may do everything possible to keep the child out of your home. Some parents will even lie; they may say that you were an abusive parent, an alcoholic—anything to make you pay for making the call. "It's like calling the cops on your daughter or son," explains attorney Ted Youmans. "You're probably not going to be befriending the kid. You'll be alienating yourself right from the start, and the system will probably treat you with alienation as the one who complained."[16]

Remember, anything that interferes with reunification is suspect, and a bad relationship between parent and grandparent is a red flag to social workers and to the courts. Judges are wary of grandparents whose children say, "I hate them. I can't get along with them. I can't visit my kids at their house; they interfere." Those grandparents may not get placement.

HOW TO AVOID INVOLVEMENT WITH THE SYSTEM

Most grandparents involved with the dependency system had no choice in the matter—a social worker showed up on their doorstep with their grandchildren in tow or the hospital held a drug-exposed infant in protective custody. In other words, the system arrived with the child. Some grandparents, however, have many chances to bypass government involvement if they realize there is a problem and know enough to think ahead.

▪ *Keep track of your grandchildren.* Do so especially when parents have problems. Offer to watch your grandchildren occasionally. Visit and call often, if the parents will let you. If there has been a problem in the past, let schools and local hospitals know that you are available as an emergency contact. Once children are in the foster care system, it can be not only difficult but heartbreaking to try to get them out.

▪ *Keep track of your adult children.* Do so even with those who don't have children yet. I have talked to grandparents from various states who tell me that they didn't even know they had a grandchild until the child was four or five years old and already in foster care. If a parent is arrested without someone available to take the child, children's services will probably take over. Keep the lines of communication open and active, especially when you're in another state. If your adult child has any responsible friends, give them your telephone number in case of emergency. Because my parents lived nearby, they were immediately able to take in my nephew when my sister died. However, had Nikki died in another city, Kevin might have gone into a foster home before anyone in the family knew it. Furthermore, since Nikki didn't have a will, child welfare might not even have known that Kevin had grandparents who could take him. The bottom line is that keeping track of the parent is the only way to keep track of the child.

▪ *Think ahead.* In case of emergency, how could you prove your relationship to your grandchild? Do you have your adult child's birth certificate? Do you have your grandchild's birth certificate? If your own child is the father, is he acknowledged on the birth certificate? If you are on good terms with the parents, in case of illness or accident, could you get a signed statement proving your relationship? Unless a grandchild is old enough to identify you, proving your relationship can be complicated, particularly if the child has a different last name from yours. Planning ahead can save time and heartache in the event of an emergency.

▪ *Consider guardianship.* If the grandchildren are with you and their parents have vanished, consider becoming their guardian. The dependency system will make you jump through legal hoops, will conduct visits once a month, and will put a social worker on your back, adding to the stress and tension you are already experiencing. But, says attorney Michael Salazar, "If you go into probate, you're on your own."[17] In other words, you're in control, not the system. (For more on guardianship, see Chapter 10.)

WHEN YOU MIGHT WANT THE SYSTEM INVOLVED

In spite of all the disadvantages, there are actually reasons you might want the system involved in your grandchild's case: the child's safety and your own peace of mind. Perhaps you cannot afford to apply for guardianship. Perhaps your family situation or personal history would prevent a judge from giving you custody. Perhaps your grandchild isn't with you, and the situation is too dangerous to wait for a guardianship hearing. This is a time when you may actually want to call child protective services. Sometimes *anything*—even foster care—is better than leaving a grandchild in an abusive home. It's not a perfect solution, but it can be the lesser evil.

Understand, however, that if you are the one to call the police or CPS, there is a possibility the child will not be placed with you. A lot depends on your background check, what your son or daughter says about you, and whether or not you live in the same state. Still, sometimes it is worth involving the system to protect a child who is at risk.

WHEN THE SYSTEM WON'T GET INVOLVED

It may seem to you that social workers and judges are just hovering in the doorways ready to snatch up any child who may be in danger, that after one call the child will be whisked away to safety. At least that is the belief of hopeful grandparents who call child abuse hotlines. Actually, it's not true. A great source of anger and frustration for many grandparents is when the system won't get involved in a case.

There are times when calling CPS won't do anything. Allegations of child abuse and neglect require witnesses and physical proof. This can infuriate grandparents who know of the kind of abuse that doesn't leave marks. Emotional abuse may not show on a child's body, but the scars are often more difficult to heal. Moreover, the legal definitions of abuse and neglect not only vary from state to state but are interpreted differently from social worker to social worker and from one judge to the next. Furthermore, leaving children with grandparents, family, or friends is rarely considered desertion or abandonment. Child welfare agencies regularly turn away children who are living with relatives without parental interference; their reasoning is that the child is not in danger.

Generally, a grandparent in this situation has three choices: continue to care for the child informally, return the child to the parents and wait until she is abused or neglected, or file for private guardianship. As we saw in Chapter 10, guardianship offers greater protection.

A WORD ABOUT SOCIAL WORKERS

In the field of social work, as in most professions, there are good workers and bad ones. Which kind you get is the luck of the draw, but the difference is often immediately clear. Good social workers are thorough. When they investigate a case, they really investigate. They talk to the children, they look for bruises and ask for explanations, they study a home for things that signal neglect. When I worked for CPS, I was sent out on a child abuse case with a social worker who never even entered the house. When Mom came to the door, he told her we had received a report of suspected child abuse. Mom said everything was fine. The social worker saw that the baby had a bottle, said okay, and left. He never looked at the other children or talked to them. This was not a good social worker.

Good social workers are supportive. They listen to your concerns, return phone calls, link you up with resources and information. They let you know what kind of financial assistance is available to your grandchild and how you can apply for it. Some will even refer you to a support group. A number of the GAP grandmothers come to me through social worker referrals.

Bad social workers are a nightmare. They range from the poorly informed to the actively heartless, from the ones who give you incorrect information about department regulations and government benefits to the ones who have a fixed prejudice against grandparents. One case worker, who didn't know me, talked to me about a grandmother I know. "She's ruining everyone's life," she told me. "I can't deal with her." She also called her "crazy" and "invasive." This attitude is a common problem for grandparents. Many social workers see them as picking fights with their children out of vengeance—"hollerin' wolf" as one grandmother calls it.[18] In fact, the war stories are legendary. I received a letter from a woman whose daughter died, leaving her with three small children to care for. Like many grandparents, she discovered that it is difficult to feed and clothe growing children on a fixed income. Her social worker told her she was expected to "cut coupons and shop at Goodwill, just like everyone else on welfare." When one young woman placed her two children with her mother, social services removed them because the grandmother was "too old." Beth and Alan Grafton had a fight on their hands to get custody of their grandchildren after their son-in-law murdered their daughter. The reason? Beth would cry when she discussed her daughter's death. The worker assigned to the case decided that Grandma "wasn't grieving properly" and recommended against custody. "The courts seem to think grandparents just love taking grandchildren from their children," says a Texas grandmother. "It's the hardest thing to do in the world. Grandparents raising grandchildren—they're not doing it because they want to, they're doing it because they have to."[19]

If you are raising your grandchildren, you will, most likely, have to work with social workers. They're like a force of nature; you can't get around them. You find them at each stage of the game, from intake workers to long-term case workers. Moreover, sometimes everything can depend on the decision of a social worker. As one young woman admitted to Claire Powers, "I look at 30 minutes in this child's life and play God." So, some words of advice . . .

▪ *Be nice to social workers.* After all, you want them on your side. Social workers have great power: They present information to judges; sometimes they're also your only source of information. Endear yourself to them, if you can. Don't make demands. "Once you attack a social worker, the likelihood of your getting satisfaction from that system is less than five percent," says attorney Michael Salazar.[20] In other words, use kid gloves and don't get them angry.

▪ *Use understanding.* It is easier to work with people if you understand what obstacles they are fighting. Social workers are as much at the mercy of an unfeeling system as are children and grandparents. Social workers in some large cities oversee as many as 125 child abuse cases.[21] They are undertrained and underpaid—and they burn out quickly. An official in one city reported that half his staff had been working less than a year.[22] Between being new on the job and having case overload, many social workers don't have time to keep up with changes in the law. Says grandparent activisit Ethel Dunn, "You go into social services [and] they are in chaos, not because everyone in the social service system is a poor social worker but it's simply that they don't have the wherewithal to do the job they're given."[23]

▪ *Tell specific facts.* Tell your grandchild's social worker what you saw with your own eyes, not what you heard from other people. If you can, offer witnesses; they may be viewed as less biased.

▪ *Consider whose case it is.* You may, as a grandparent, talk about "my case" and "my social worker," and it can certainly feel that way. You are trying to protect your grandchild from parents and a system that seem to have anything but your grandchild's best interests at heart. Grandparents have a lot riding on their social worker and their case. A good social worker may understand this, but he won't see it the same way. He can't. He is your grandchild's social worker, handling your grandchild's case. His job is to protect the child's interests and, if possible, return her to the custody of her parents.

Remember, not every social worker who disagrees with a grandparent is a bad social worker. Not every child who cannot be with his parents should be with his grandparents. There are grandparents who really should not have their grandchildren because of health, medical, or psychological problems. Some children may be better off in a foster home if there is no other relative to take them.

A WORD ABOUT JUDGES

The judge is the wild card in any legal situation. Judges don't write laws, but they interpret them. Judges don't investigate cases, but they rule on them. In a limited time frame and with selective information a judge makes binding decisions about a child's future, and each decision is as individual as the judge who made it. Judges get reputations among grandparents. Some judges are rule-bound. "They're lawyers," says attorney Charles Ollinger. "They are taught to think unemotionally, to think about 'best interest' in legal terms. The good ones listen to people who understand emotional realities—psychologists, child care professionals—but there aren't many judges like that."[24]

Some judges can seem terribly unfair and inconsistent. Like the one who let nine-year-old Travis Jackson testify against his father for killing his mother but wouldn't let him choose to live with his grandparents. Or the judge who sent Esther Smith's grandsons back to an alcoholic mother who had not complied with her case plan because he felt the case had been in the system "long enough." Others are plainly insensitive. "Some grandparents have a need to steal their grandchildren," one judge told a grandmother. "Is that the case here?" I have even heard about a probate judge who turned to an attorney and barked, "What's all this about 'bonding?' We're not talking about real estate here!"

Every once in a while we hear about a judge who not only is sensitive to grandparents' and grandchildren's interests but understands what is at stake. One unorthodox judge in Arizona settled a dispute in which everyone in a large family was fighting bitterly over two grandchildren. The judge had every person involved in the case come into the courtroom and forbade anyone to speak. Then she had the children brought in. She watched to see whom they ran to—it turned out to be the grandparents—and awarded them custody.[25]

For the most part, however, few judges even think about grandparent concerns, let alone support them. Part of the reason is that they often cannot. Judges interpret the laws but they are limited by them, and according to the law, reunification of child and parent has the highest priority. "I can't take a child from a parent because I'd like to," says California Judge John C. Woolley. "I can't even take a child from a parent because down deep in my heart I really want to. I can only interfere in a parent–child relationship if to continue that relationship would be a detriment to the child and further to place the child with a nonparent is in the child's best interest. It's not a balancing act; it's a dual-focus question."[26]

Another problem, however, is that judges, like social workers, have impossible caseloads. They may not have time to read all the critical documents involved in a case, and they may come to court unprepared. Their decisions can reflect that.

If you find yourself in the dependency system or if you apply for guardianship or adoption or even if you appeal an administrative decision about government aid, you may find yourself facing a judge. If you do and you are given the opportunity to speak in court, there are a few principles you may want to keep in mind:

▪ *Be respectful.*
▪ *Be clear.* Make your statements short and to the point. Stick to facts. Ask the judge if he or she has any questions.
▪ *Be informed.* There are some situations in which grandparents may represent themselves in court, such as in visitation or guardianship hearings in certain states. If you are in such a situation, you are

expected to be as familiar with the laws and procedures that affect your case as an attorney is. If you represent yourself, educate yourself.

▪ *Don't argue with the judge.* It is particularly critical to follow this rule before a decision is reached. "It is," says Ollinger, "like arguing with a waiter before the waiter brings the soup. You don't know what is going to happen!"[27]

No two courtrooms are the same. Everything that happens in a particular courtroom is filtered through the perpective of the presiding judge. Which judge you get is often the luck of the draw. Unfortunately, it can set the tone for your granchild's entire case.

CHAPTER 12

Government Aid and Public Assistance

Just when you think you should be living the life
of Riley, you've got a whole new family. I spend
at least $80 every week on groceries; if it was
just the two of us, it would be half of that.
—*Grandmother in North Carolina*[1]

R aising a grandchild is not only an emotional
and legal challenge but a financial one as well.
Some grandparents deplete their savings,
take out second mortgages on their homes, and even do without
their own necessities in order to provide for their grandchildren. Few
think about government aid. Many grandparents simply don't know
that financial assistance is available to them; often this is because
they have their grandchildren on an informal basis. However, even
when children are placed by child protective services or the court,
many social workers neglect to tell grandparents and relatives that
they are entitled to aid for a child.

Remember Leah Croft? She was already raising her daughter's
six-year-old twins when another grandchild, Josh, arrived at her
house—late at night, unexpected, and in the arms of a social worker.
Leah was a single, working grandmother on a moderate salary. The
twins had lived with her for four years, and she had stretched her
limited budget to accommodate them. She didn't know the twins
were entitled to welfare benefits, so she had never asked for them.
Then the new baby arrived, and the expenses nearly took her over the
financial edge. Although Josh was placed with her by child protective
services, no one from the agency told her that he might be eligible

for foster care. Furthermore, after Leah found out and applied for foster care, no one told her she could get welfare assistance for the baby while she waited. For five months she put diapers and baby supplies on her credit card, because that was all she had. Leah eventually received retroactive benefits for the months she waited, but she is still paying the interest those credit card charges incurred.

Lack of information is the toughest financial problem you may face as a grandparent; it keeps you out of the game entirely. If you don't know you can't ask, and if you can't ask you may not get the help you need and deserve. The good news is that government assistance is available to you, primarily through programs that support dependent children. Just because you are caring for your grandchildren does not mean you have an obligation to support them—even if you are their legal guardian. Only parents (biological or adoptive) have that responsibility. The government recognizes this, which is why programs like foster care were developed. Although grandparents fall into a gray area between parents and foster parents, there are a number of assistance programs that may apply to you and your grandchildren, from welfare and foster care benefits to social security and adoption assistance.

THE DIFFICULTIES OF WORKING WITH THE GOVERNMENT

Government aid means working with the government. You may find yourself fighting a maze of bureaucracy, poor information, and seemingly unfair rules. You may also struggle with the social stigma of welfare or the inequalities of the foster care system. The very agencies designed to support your grandchildren can seem like more of a hindrance than a help. Be aware of the pitfalls. Advanced knowledge can often prevent problems, and it will always prepare you to face them.

Misinformation

After lack of information, the most common problem grandparents face in dealing with government agencies is poor information. You may ask the right questions, but the answers you get are either half true or completely wrong. The reason is that many social and welfare workers just don't know the right answers. They may be undertrained or unaware of changes in the law. Perhaps they don't understand how a particular program applies to grandparent families. For instance, you yourself may not be eligible for welfare, but your grandchild may be. But if no one tells you, you won't know.

Government employees are rarely malicious but may be ill informed. Unfortunately, some of them will swear their poor information is the gospel truth. Be cautious when you deal with social workers and eligibility workers. Ask questions to clarify what they tell you. Learn what you can about local rules and regulations, and contact other grandparents and support groups to compare notes. Accurate information is your key to government assistance.

Bureaucracy

Dealing with government agencies is rarely a cut-and-dry experience. It can mean long lines, extensive paperwork, and bureaucratic mistakes. You may wait in three different lines at the welfare office just to get a packet of forms, then wait in another line to schedule an appointment. If you work, you may have to take the day off in order to attend an interview. If your grandchildren have to be there, you'll need to cart toys and lunch along for them. It could turn into a whole day affair. This is particularly difficult for grandparents who are disabled and cannot sit for long periods of time. Calling isn't better. Because some eligibility workers have restricted telephone hours, it can take days to connect with them.

If you are having a difficult time reaching an eligibility worker, you may want to talk to her supervisor. First, document the times you try to call and the names of people you speak with. Write letters when you can (and keep copies for yourself). Then, if you do have to go over the worker's head, you have proof of what occurred.

Long lines and mistakes are an inevitable part of dealing with the government. All you can do is be alert for errors and be patient with the rest—and try to do something nice for yourself when you get home!

Unequal Benefits

There are two key assistance programs that grandparents and relatives get involved with: welfare (Aid to Families with Dependent Children, or AFDC) and foster care. Both provide cash and medical assistance to needy children, but foster care offers substantially higher benefits. In one year the average (national) welfare payment to a grandparent who was the sole caregiver for a grandchild was $109 per child per month, compared to $371 per child per month to foster parents.[2] Foster care also increases with the child's age and may include respite care and clothing vouchers. Grandparents may receive foster care benefits for a grandchild but only if that child is a dependent of the juvenile court system and meets selected criteria (see "Foster Care," below). This means that of children who are abused and abandoned by their parents and living with grandparents, only those placed by court order may be eligible for the higher benefits.

In many states, unrelated foster parents are also entitled to additional benefits and services that may not be available to family members.

One reason for the inequality, according to children's rights advocates, is that society expects families to take care of their children. Foster care benefits only provide for children who become the responsibility of the state. However, notes the *Washington Post*," Child welfare laws were written before the crack epidemic, which made the extended family a critical response to lack of care by parents."[3]

It is a sad fact that government programs designed to help children who have been abused or abandoned by their parents don't always support keeping those children in families. Some grandparents live at the poverty level and can barely afford to raise grandchildren even with help from welfare. They may find themselves sliding into debt or even surrendering their grandchildren to the dependency system and the care of unrelated foster parents.

One couple in Missouri took in five grandchildren when their son and daughter-in-law lost custody. The grandfather makes $23,000 per year, and Grandma stays home with the kids. Each month they receive only $384 in welfare benefits for the care and feeding of five growing children. They cannot get food stamps because Grandpa makes too much money. "We are now behind in our bills," he writes. "Our utilities are about to get cut off, and we can't seem to make ends meet. We don't want to send these children to a foster home, but with these financial problems, we are almost forced to send them to one." Had these children qualified for foster care, the family would have received at least $900 a month, an average of $180 per child.[4] To quote one grandmother in Cleveland, "No one can tell you you're raising your grandchild for money!"

Social Stigma

Perhaps the hardest thing about asking for help is the social stigma. Too many people think welfare is synonymous with being lazy instead of needy, and that attitude can be reflected by many state employees. Grandparents often receive scorn rather than sympathy when they take in a grandchild and need to seek aid. Some grandparents don't look like they need assistance and are made to feel guilty about asking for it. There are eligibility workers who act as if they're pulling money out of their own pockets. "You do walk on eggshells when you deal with social services," says Ada MacKenzie. "Those people talk to you like they talk to a dog."

Grandparents who get foster care benefits have it slightly easier. They don't have to sit in line at the welfare office to talk to eligibility workers. Because they are taking over for the state, they are treated more like Good Samaritans than welfare recipients—although the only difference between the two might be a call to child protective services.

This kind of prejudice, like bureaucracy, is a frustrating reality of government assistance. You can try to ignore it. You can air out your feelings in a support group or with other grandparents. But try not to let it eat away at you; it will only drain you of the energy you need to raise your grandchildren. The truth is, every grandparent who takes a child is doing something wonderful for society. If these kids went to the state, the state would be putting out a lot more money and resources to care for them.

Don't be discouraged. These programs exist to help children in need. If your grandchildren qualify for them, they deserve the assistance. And you deserve the financial relief. Even if what you get from welfare isn't enough to raise a child, it still helps, and every bit of help counts. A few hundred dollars can make a great difference to a grandparent struggling on a fixed income, and the medical assistance can be a lifesaver if you cannot put your grandchildren on your insurance policy.

The rest of this chapter looks at federal assistance programs one by one. It discusses what they are, what you get, what you need to qualify for them, and what you as a grandparent need to know to receive the most help. Each program description is only a blueprint of what you may encounter. Although these are federally sponsored programs, they are administered by state, county, and local governments, and their regulations and benefits often vary. Also, many of these programs are subject to change whenever welfare and health care reforms take effect. So, consider this chapter a primer; it offers enough information to spark questions. Then check local resources for current, detailed information about the implementation of federal assistance programs in your state. Remember, the more information you have, the better armed you are to work the system—instead of being worked over by the system.

AID TO FAMILIES WITH DEPENDENT CHILDREN (AFDC)

What It Is

AFDC is the major child welfare program in the United States. It is designed to provide needy children and their families with monthly cash assistance to help pay for basic needs like food, clothing, and rent. Although the federal government sets general AFDC guidelines, each state sets its own definition of neediness, establishes its own income limits and benefit levels, and administers the program. The actual funds for AFDC come from a combination of federal, state, and, occasionally, county sources. A majority of AFDC recipients are single women with children, but the program applies to any close family member who cares for low-income children.

Who Is Eligible

In order to qualify for AFDC a child must fulfill three major requirements: He must be a (1) deprived of parental support, (2) living with a relative caretaker, and (3) poor or financially needy. In most instances, if you are raising your grandchild, he is eligible for AFDC benefits. But let's look at the requirements one at a time:

Deprived of Parental Support

The government considers children deprived, or dependent, if they are living without the support of one parent because that parent is dead, missing, disabled, or unemployed. Most children who live with their grandparents are deprived of parental support.

Living with a Relative Caretaker

If you are a grandparent and your grandchild is living in your home, you are by definition a relative caretaker.

Poor or Financially Needy

In order to be financially eligible for AFDC, the income and resources of the child's "family unit" must be below certain federal and state limits. An AFDC family unit is basically the parent(s) of a dependent child, the child, and any dependent brothers or sisters in the home.

Only the income of the child, the parents, and the siblings can be used to determine financial need and only if they live in the same house. The income of parents who do not live with or help support a child does not count toward the child's AFDC grant (although the government may go after the parents for reimbursement or child support). Nor can your income affect your grandchild's application. Unless your grandchildren have their own regular source of income, they will probably qualify as needy.

Relative caretakers, even guardians, have no legal responsibility to financially support a child, and your finances cannot be considered. The exception is if you yourself are in financial need and want to apply for aid *with* your grandchild; in that case, your income and resources will be taken into consideration (although your home, furniture, and most personal possessions will not be).

Miscellaneous Requirements

There are also several additional requirements your grandchild must satisfy before she can receive AFDC. The child must be a U.S. citizen or legal permanent resident of the United States and a legal resident of your state. She must also be under 18 (under 19 if a full-time student) and have a valid Social Security number. If there are any other rules that apply to your family, your grandchild's caseworker should be able to explain them to you.

What You Get

Those who receive AFDC get monthly cash benefits, medical assistance, and, occasionally, food stamps. The amount of money a family can receive depends on the number of people in the family unit and on the amount and source of income. Benefits vary from state to state and sometimes from county to county. For example, in 1990 a two-person family (presumably parent and child) could have received $88 a month in Alabama, $274 in Ohio, $560 in California, and as much as $752 in Alaska. The national median that year was $294 for a family of two.[5]

Medical assistance is the second part of AFDC benefits. Families receiving AFDC are automatically entitled to Medicaid or to their state's equivalent. However, many children who don't qualify for AFDC may still qualify for Medicaid; make sure you ask about it for your grandchild (see "Medicaid," later in this chapter).

Many AFDC families are also eligible to receive food stamps. While a grandparent's income cannot be considered for AFDC eligibility, it is counted for food stamps. Thus, it is possible that you could receive AFDC for your grandchildren but not qualify for food stamps. Even so, it is worth a try. (See "Food Stamps," below.)

The Application Process

How It Should Work

You can apply for AFDC at your state or local welfare office. Call ahead to confirm office hours and make sure you have the right office for your area. Find out if you need an appointment or if you can just come in. (See "What You Need to Bring," below.)

To apply for AFDC you must file a written application and pass income and resources tests. The welfare office has a responsibility to help you with your application and to help you get the documentation you need.[6] My experience has been that they don't often do this, but they should. If you run into problems, contact your Legal Aid office.

Your application should be processed within 45 days. If aid is denied, the denial must be in writing. If you feel this decision was unfair, you can request a "fair hearing." The written denial usually explains how to do this.

Once you begin to receive AFDC, you must make monthly reports about your grandchild's income (and about yours if you applied with your grandchild). The amount of the benefits will be determined month to month, based on each month's circumstances. You will also face a periodic "redetermination," a process in which the welfare department reviews each family's eligibility as if it were a new application.

What You Need to Bring

When you go for your intake interview, try to take as many records as possible to prove your grandchild's eligibility (and yours, if you are applying with your grandchild). Make sure you have photocopies for the application. Never give away your originals. Don't panic if you can't put your hands on everything; it is the responsibility of the welfare office to reasonably help you get all the required documentation.

To apply for AFDC for your grandchild, you will need the following:

- Proof of the child's age and identity, for example, a birth certificate (few grandparents actually have their grandchild's birth certificate, but you can request a copy from the county where your grandchild was born).
- Proof of the child's residence, for example, school records or a letter to the address.
- The child's Social Security number.
- Proof of your tie to the child (the parent's birth certificate, along with the child's birth certificate, should establish your relationship).
- Proof of income of the child.
- Proof of the child's citizenship or immigration status.

The welfare office cannot limit you to a particular form of identification or proof. For instance, if you cannot find a birth certificate, you should be able to use another proof of age or identity.

▪ WHAT YOU NEED TO KNOW

There is great confusion out there about how grandparents apply for aid for their grandchildren and how aid is determined. Many eligibility workers are used to dealing with regular parent–child applications. They just don't know how the laws and regulations affect grandparents, and they often give out information that is simply *wrong*. The following paragraphs discuss some critical issues grandparents need to understand:

▪ *Your income doesn't count.* One of the biggest problems a grandparent faces with an AFDC application is answering the questions about income. These are equally baffling to eligibility workers, who may give out the wrong information and often count Grandma's income when they shouldn't.

I cannot emphasize this enough: Unless you are applying for AFDC *with* your grandchild or you have adopted your grandchild, your income does not count. You are considered a "non-needy caretaker" and you are filling out the application for your grandchild, not for yourself.[7] Despite what they tell you, fill out the form *as if you were the child.* For instance, if the question is "Do you own a home?," the answer is no (you may own a home, but the child does not). If the question is "Do you have a bank account?," the answer is no if the child does not have a bank account. It doesn't matter what your income and circumstances are; your grandchild is eligible for AFDC. This is true even if you become a legal guardian. If you fill out the forms based on *your* income, the application will be denied. That is exactly what happened to Janet Baker when she was given the wrong information at the welfare office. Not only did they turn her down, but they made her feel awful for even daring to ask for help. "It was three months before I finally got some assistance for the children," says Janet. "By that time, our financial situation was even worse. I felt really battered. The process of finding out just how to do that was a major step for me. I felt degraded."

According to Yolanda Vera, staff attorney for the National Health Law Program, there are only three situations in which your income can be counted in the AFDC application: If you have adopted your grandchild, if you are applying for aid *with* your grandchild, or if you are reaching into your pockets and giving the child money every month. But, says Vera, "If you say, 'I love my grandchild, but I don't expect to support her,' then they cannot count your resources or income, even if you are a Rockefeller."[8]

▪ *You can apply for AFDC for yourself.* If you are raising an AFDC-eligible child and you yourself meet the criteria for welfare benefits, you may apply with your grandchild as a family unit. Even if your grandchild receives Supplemental Security Income (SSI) or foster care (see below), he may still qualify your family for AFDC, although he won't count toward the amount of assistance you receive.[9]

■ *Immediate aid is possible.* Families who don't have enough to meet their basic living needs may be eligible for "AFDC Immediate Need Cash," a program that is partially funded by the federal government. If you qualify, the agency should speed up your AFDC application and advance your first AFDC check within a few days. You can apply for Immediate Need Cash when you apply for AFDC, but you may have to push for information about it. Although Immediate Need Cash (or its equivalent) is available in some states, it is not often discussed, at least not with grandparents. Try to take as many documents as possible to show that you qualify.

■ *You should keep records.* Papers get lost and conversations forgotten. Remember to keep copies of all the documents you turn in to any welfare office. Also, keep track of all conversations you have and all attempted contacts with agency personnel. If you can, send letters that confirm any information you receive, and keep copies of those letters. If your information is incorrect, the agency should write back and correct it. If not, you have it confirmed in writing.[10] This could be useful if you ever have to appeal.

■ *You can appeal.* If your application is denied or your benefits are discontinued, you must be notified in writing. If you feel that your benefits have been denied or discontinued unfairly or that you are not receiving the correct amount of benefits or that you are being mistreated by a welfare worker, you have the right to request a state hearing. Although this can be done by filling out a hearing request form or making a phone call, the most efficient way to request a hearing is to fill out the form on the back of your denial notice. Photocopy both sides of the notice for your records before you return it.

■ *You may want to get legal representation.* If you do appeal, it can be helpful to have an advocate or an attorney handle your case. Grandparents who cannot afford counsel can sometimes find pro bono or discounted help through organizations like Legal Aid or welfare rights groups. The Legal Aid Foundation of Los Angeles has helped some of our grandparents appeal government decisions and receive aid they could not get on their own.

■ *You might lose AFDC to unscrupulous parents.* Many parents are manipulative and know how to use the system to their advantage. I can't begin to tell you how many cases I know of in which parents continue to receive AFDC although they are no longer supporting their children. This is illegal. AFDC money is there for the care of needy children. If Mom or Dad continues to take the checks when you are raising the child, they may be guilty of fraud.

However, grandparents who lack legal custody often won't make waves about AFDC; they are too fearful that Mom or Dad will turn around and take the child back in order to get the benefits. Even when grandparents do make waves, not much may happen. I know grandparents who have repeatedly reported the parents for fraud, and nothing has changed; they still have their grandchildren, and the parents continue to receive AFDC.

FOSTER CARE AND YOUAKIM

What It Is

Foster care benefits—properly known as federal IV-E (four-E) foster care—are a type of AFDC benefits for children who have been removed from their homes by child protective services and are living somewhere else.[11] "Youakim" (pronounced "yo-kim") benefits are federal foster care benefits in cases where a child has been placed with a relative. Some areas also have state and county foster care programs, which may not apply to relatives.

The name Youakim refers to a 1979 lawsuit, *Miller v. Youakim*, in which the U.S. Supreme Court ruled that children who are placed by court order cannot be denied foster care benefits because they had been placed in the home of a relative.[12] Before 1979 only nonrelatives could get foster care benefits. Every state participating in the federal program should offer these benefits, although not every state refers to federal relative foster care assistance as Youakim. (If your state child welfare agency does not recognize the term *Youakim*, ask for federal relative or family foster care. For simplicity's sake, in this chapter we will use the term *Youakim*.)

Who Is Eligible

For your grandchild to qualify for federal foster care or Youakim, she must fulfill three general requirements: she must be (1) a dependent of the court, (2) AFDC-eligible and AFDC-linked, and (3) in an approved placement. These requirements get confusing, particularly since states vary on their interpretations of the law, so let's look at them one at a time:

Dependent of the Court

To be a dependent of the court your grandchild must have been removed from her parents, other relatives, or legal guardian and placed with you by a juvenile court order. If you have taken your grandchild into your home or if child welfare placed the child with you without a court order, she will not be eligible for Youakim.

AFDC-Eligible and AFDC-Linked

AFDC-eligible simply means that your grandchild fulfills the major requirements for AFDC eligibility—that is, he is deprived of parental support, needy, and living with a relative—as well as the additional requirements of age, residence, citizenship, and a social security number.

AFDC-linked is more complicated. This is the requirement that is most open to interpretation and confusion. According to federal law, AFDC linkage means any one of the following three things:

1. The child was receiving AFDC in the month the child welfare agency petitioned for his removal.
2. The child could have received AFDC if the parent had applied in the month of the court petition.
3. The child was living with a relative for six months before the petition was filed and could have received AFDC with that relative.

The question of whether a child *could have* received AFDC centers on the child's financial situation in the month he was removed. If the child was removed from his parent's home, the parent's income should count toward AFDC eligibility. The difficulty with this requirement is that in order to determine if the child was eligible you often need to talk to the parent who had custody if you need information about the parent's finances. Unfortunately, the parent may not be around or may be too angry or too high to be helpful. If the parent is available and cooperative, getting this information is not a problem. If the parent was receiving welfare at that time, it is also not a problem, since the welfare office has access to those records. But if he or she is missing or uncooperative, you could have a tough time meeting this requirement.

Another problem with linkage is that while federal law says one thing, states often pass regulations that say something else, sometimes creating policies that are more restrictive than federal requirements. This means that children who are eligible for family foster care under federal law could still be denied federal benefits because of individual state regulations.[13] If your grandchild meets your state requirements for AFDC linkage, you don't have a problem. If he doesn't meet state requirements, but meets federal requirements you can request a hearing.

Approved Placement

The last requirement for federal foster care assistance, and for Youakim, is that the child be in an approved placement. That means the child is placed in the home of a relative approved by the child welfare agency or in a licensed foster care facility.

What You Get

Foster care benefits include monthly cash benefits, health care services through Medicaid, and some additional social services. Foster care benefits are higher than AFDC because foster children are presumed to have greater needs than children on welfare. Unlike AFDC, where benefits are determined by family size, foster care and Youakim are based on the age and needs of each child. In many areas, special needs children—those who are developmentally delayed, physically challenged, prenatally drug exposed, and so on—may also be entitled to additional benefits called "specialized care rates." These rates increase the amount of a child's foster care grant. However, states vary according to the specialized rates they provide and the eligibility requirements for them. If you think your grandchild qualifies for specialized care rates, talk to the social worker. If the child qualifies, you may be required to attend a short training course about handling those special needs.

Foster children automatically qualify for Medicaid and may also be eligible for certain social services, including a clothing allowance, free school breakfast and lunch, and, occasionally, respite care. However, both the dollar amount of Youakim benefits and the scope of health care coverage and services vary state by state, and sometimes even within individual states.

Youakim continues until a child's 18th birthday. In some states benefits can continue until the child is 19 as long as the child remains in foster care; continues to meet financial eligibility requirements; and continues to attend a high school, vocational, or technical school full-time and expects to finish by her 19th birthday.

Although Youakim benefits only address the needs of the dependent child, you may be able to apply for AFDC for yourself while you receive foster care benefits for your grandchild if you are financially needy.

The Application Process

How It Should Work

The children's services worker should be the one to start the application process for you. Once the child has been removed by child protection and placed with you by court order, the children's services worker is supposed to explain your benefit choices, which in most cases is either AFDC or Youakim (if the child qualifies).

For many grandparents, choosing between AFDC and foster care benefits (Youakim) can be something of a gamble. It is easier to qualify for AFDC, but Youakim benefits are higher. If you go with AFDC but your grandchild was eligible for Youakim, you lose the higher benefits. On the other hand, if you choose Youakim and a month later discover that your grandchild doesn't qualify, you will have lost a month of AFDC benefits. You can apply for AFDC while you are waiting for a foster care decision (see "What You Need to Know," below.)

Once you decide, the worker should either help you collect the information you need to establish the child's eligibility for Youakim or, if you choose AFDC, process your grandchild's AFDC application. He should also explain your foster care rights and responsibilities and immediately obtain a Medicaid card for your grandchild.

How It Often Works

Unfortunately, social workers often neglect to explain government benefits to relative caregivers. I have had grandparents call me months, and even years, after a child was placed with them by the court, and they hadn't even known the child was eligible for benefits and Medicaid.

▪ WHAT YOU NEED TO KNOW

▪ *Youakim is a court-related program.* To be eligible for Youakim your grandchildren must be placed in your home by a court order. If the parents just leave them with you or if you take them in informally, they will not be eligible for these benefits: If for example, your granddaughter calls and tells you that Mom has been sleeping for two days and there is no food in the house. If you simply pick her up and never involve the courts, she will not qualify for Youakim. If, on the other hand, you call a social worker and make a referral of neglect *and* if child protective services removes the child *and* if Mom was eligible for AFDC and signs the necessary papers, or was already receiving it, then the child should be eligible for federal foster care benefits.

The problem is that most grandparents won't leave children in a neglectful situation in the hopes that a social worker will get there in time. They will rush in to rescue their grandchildren—and end up paying for it in the pocket. Foster care is related to court placement, and the courts only get involved when a child is in danger. If you have the child and the parent is not an immediate threat to her safety, the child welfare system may consider the child well protected and refuse to open a case. One social worker told a grandmother that the only way to become a foster parent would be to abandon her grandchildren, have them placed in foster care, and then apply for custody. Of course, Grandma knew that there was no guarantee that she would actually get the children and that in the meantime they ran the risk of being further traumatized. Grandma stayed with lower benefits.[14]

▪ *You can apply for AFDC and foster care assistance at the same time.* Relatives are sometimes told they can apply for either AFDC or foster care, but not both. They are also told that once they make a choice and benefits start, they cannot change their minds. Neither of these statements is true. While you cannot receive duplicate aid for the same child in the same period, nothing in the law prevents you from applying for both, especially if there is a chance that the child might not qualify for Youakim. You can also start on AFDC and then switch to Youakim, if your grandchild qualifies.

Unfortunately, each approach has its disadvantages: If you only apply for Youakim and are approved, your grandchild will receive the higher benefits dating back to the day you applied. If, instead, you apply for both and receive AFDC while you wait for Youakim approval, you will lose those retroactive benefits. On the other hand, if you only apply for Youakim and are eventually denied, your grandchild will have gone several months without any benefits at all. This is particularly hard on lower-income grandparents who not only need the higher benefits but also need immediate help.

■ *You can appeal.* If your grandchild does not qualify for Youakim benefits and if you dispute that decision, you can request a state hearing.

■ *Guardianship generally eliminates Youakim.* Social workers often encourage grandparents to become the legal guardians of their grandchildren without explaining the full economic impact of this decision. But becoming a guardian can sharply affect your financial situation, especially if you are raising your grandchild on a limited income. To receive foster care payments, a child must be a dependent of the court. Once you become your grandchild's guardian, that dependency ends and so does the child's eligibility for the higher Youakim benefits. He may still qualify for AFDC, but it will mean less money and, possibly, fewer services.

Rebecca Tybor is a grandmother who has her grandchildren with her in long-term foster care. Applying for guardianship would give her much more control in her granddaughters' lives. Right now, if she wants to take the kids on a trip, she may have to consult the courts; as guardian, she would have free rein. But she can't afford to lose the benefits she has with Youakim, so she stays "married" to the child welfare system. There is one exception to this dilemma: If the judge who rules on your guardianship states in her order that "the placement and care of the child remain the responsibility of the Department of Social Services" (42 U.S.C. Section 672), you may still be eligible for foster care benefits.[15] If you cannot do without the child's foster care benefits, ask the judge to insert this language into the guardianship order. However, you will continue to have child welfare involved in your grandchild's case.

SUPPLEMENTAL SECURITY INCOME (SSI) FOR CHILDREN

What It Is

Like AFDC, SSI is a federal cash assistance program for people in need. But while AFDC is designed to help children who are poor and deprived, SSI assists those who are poor and blind or disabled. Also,

SSI typically offers higher benefits than AFDC and does not automatically end at 18. Children who continue to meet SSI financial and disability requirements may continue to receive benefits into adulthood.

Who Is Eligible

Two factors determine SSI eligibility for children under 18: financial need and disability. Your grandchild must fill both requirements to qualify for SSI benefits.

Financial Need

With SSI, as with AFDC, financial need is based on the income and assets of the child, not the guardian. Your financial situation should not affect your grandchild's application. However, SSI will count any AFDC, Youakim, or adoption assistance benefits your grandchild receives, as well as Social Security Survivors Benefits (see below). Each state sets its own eligibility limits, within federal guidelines, for income and resources.

Disability

For SSI purposes, children are considered disabled if they have a physical or mental condition that is as severe as one that would prevent an adult from working. In other words, the condition keeps them from doing things and behaving in ways that are normal for other children of the same age, such as holding their head steady at three months or walking by 20 months. This disability must also be one that is expected to last at least 12 months or result in the child's death. Social Security regulations include a specific list of conditions that qualify as disabilities. If your grandchild's condition is not on that list or not equal to a condition on that list, eligibility will be determined by her ability to function in everyday life.

What You Get

Children who qualify for SSI receive cash assistance and health care services through Medicaid and Children with Special Health Care Needs (CSHCN) programs.

Monthly Cash Benefits

How much cash assistance your grandchild receives depends on where you live, since many states supplement the federal program with state funding.

Health Care Services

In addition to Medicaid, SSI children are entitled to additional health care services under the Children with Special Health Care Needs (CSHCN) provisions of the Social Security Act. CSHCN programs are usually administered by state health agencies. The names and regulations of these programs vary from state to state, but most offer specialized services through private doctors, clinics, hospitals, and community agencies. A child who is not eligible for cash assistance through SSI may still be eligible for medical assistance through a local CSHCN program. Check with your local health department, social services office, or hospital for more information.

The Application Process

How It Should Work

You can apply for SSI by calling the Social Security Administration (SSA) and scheduling an interview with your local Social Security office. The SSA will then send you forms to be completed before the interview and to be filed with your application.

Once you apply, the local Social Security office will decide whether your grandchild's income and assets/resources are within federal and state SSI limits. Then all the information about your grandchild's medical condition will be sent to a state agency, usually called the Disability Determination Service (DDS), for review by a disability evaluation specialist and a doctor. The DDS team will look at how your grandchild's condition affects her functioning in everyday life to decide if she meets the SSI criteria for disability. To do this, they will consider both medical evidence and nonmedical evidence (i.e., letters from teachers, doctors, child care providers, etc.). If your grandchild does not have thorough medical records, you may be asked to take the child for a special exam that Social Security will pay for.[16]

How It Often Works

It is not uncommon for the Social Security Administration to take more than six months to decide SSI eligibility, and even then many cases are incorrectly denied, often owing to a lack of medical or psychiatric documentation. However, many denials are overturned on appeal. If your grandchild is denied, you have a legal right to appeal the decision. If the appeal is successful, he may even receive retroactive benefits based upon the date of the original application.

What You Need to Bring

The more information you bring to your SSI appointment, the easier it will be for Social Security to process your grandchild's application. You will need two kinds of documentation for your grandchild's SSI application: records that show income eligibility and those that confirm the child's disability.

To show your grandchild's income eligibility, you will need to bring the child's

- Social Security number
- Birth certificate or other proof of age
- Financial records and other information about the child's income and resources
- Proof of citizenship or immigration status (birth certificate, green card, visa, passport, immigration papers, etc.)

To prove your grandchild's disability, you must describe, in as much detail as possible, how the disability prevents him from doing things that other children of the same age can normally do. Just because a child is born drug exposed, for instance, is not enough to qualify him as disabled. While some children are indeed severely disabled from prenatal drug exposure, others seem to function normally. DDS needs thorough, detailed information. Records that can help include:

▪ *Medical records.* Bring information on *all* medical problems, past and present, that the child has experienced. Even problems that seem unrelated to the disability could be important. In fact, to avoid forgetting anything in the interview, you might consider making a list of all the reasons you think your grandchild is disabled.

■ *List of medical personnel.* Bring the names, addresses, and phone numbers of all doctors, hospitals, clinics, and specialists who have treated the child. Be as specific as possible. If you can, provide dates of visits and medical account numbers to help get records as soon as possible.

■ *Nonmedical records.* Social Security doesn't just use medical evidence to decide a child's eligibility for SSI. The agency also considers evidence that shows whether a child can do "age-appropriate activities." Since the disability examiner is not able to see the child, he has to rely on reports from nonmedical sources about what the child can and cannot do and how she manages everyday tasks. Helpful nonmedical records include school records; special education or early intervention plans, if the child has one (see Chapter 13); the names and addresses of teachers, therapists, social workers, child care providers, clergy, relatives, and neighbors who can describe the child's ability to perform everyday activities.

■ *Letters with specific examples.* If possible, ask all your medical and nonmedical sources to provide you with written reports about your grandchild in addition to their standard records. Ask them—as well as family members and clergy—to describe in detail how the disability interferes with the child's everyday activities and to give specific examples. Write down your own observations about your grandchild's disability as well.

Don't wait to have all your paperwork together before you apply. Although it can take months to decide whether your grandchild qualifies for SSI, the payments will go back to the date of your initial visit or phone call as long as the application is filed within the following 60 days.[17] The Social Security staff is supposed to help you find missing documents or suggest substitutes, and many communities have special arrangements between medical providers, social service agencies, and schools.

■ WHAT YOU NEED TO KNOW

■ *You don't have to mail original documents.* Although the Social Security Administration requires original documents to process your application, you can take them into your local Social Security office in person and they can make the copies they need and immediately return your originals.

▪ *It's important to get things in writing.* Anything government workers tell you about your case—instructions or changes—ask them to put it in writing. Also, keep copies of anything you send to government offices. On the copy, mark the date you mailed the letter.

▪ *Your grandchild's doctor can do the evaluation.* SSI decides most cases on the basis of medical assessments. A child has a right to have evidence submitted by her own doctor and to have that individual conduct the follow-up assessments as well. If there is a need for additional testing, Social Security should pay for it, whether the agency uses your grandchild's physician or its own.[18]

▪ *There are special cases.* Although Social Security can take several months to evaluate whether a child is disabled, there are exceptions. Individuals whose condition is so severe that they are automatically presumed to be disabled can receive SSI benefits for up to six months while the formal disability decision is being made. These conditions include, but are not limited to, HIV infection; blindness; Down syndrome; and some cases of deafness, cerebral palsy, and muscular dystrophy.[19]

▪ *Cash gifts to your grandchild will count against the SSI benefits.* According to attorney Pamela Mohr, if you want to give the child a gift or start a college fund, do it as a "blocked trust" account that he or she cannot access; otherwise, it may count as income.

▪ *SSA must be notified about changes.* Once your grandchild gets SSI, you must notify SSA about any change in his address, income, medical condition, living arrangements, and school attendance. The agency must be notified if he leaves the United States. If you do not report these changes on time, your grandchild could lose his SSI eligibility.

▪ *It is important to keep receipts.* SSI is only for the daily support of the eligible child, and you must account for this money every year. If you spend it on anything else, such as a college fund, Social Security could require you to pay it back.[20]

▪ *SSA can send SSI checks to your bank.* In some cases it is possible to have SSI checks deposited directly to your bank account, if you have one. If you can do this, it is the safest way to handle your grandchild's benefits. However, it is still important to keep detailed records of how this money is spent.

▪ *During the appeal process, your grandchild may still be eligible for AFDC and Medicaid.* Appealing an SSI denial can be a long process, and you won't receive benefits for your grandchild during the course of it. If you do appeal an SSI denial, see if you can apply for AFDC and Medicaid in the meantime.

▪ *You may want to get legal assistance.* The appeal process can be long and complicated. It can be helpful to have an attorney or advocate in your camp. If you can't afford an attorney, your local Legal Aid office may be able to help you. If your grandchild is developmentally delayed or mentally ill, you may be able to get legal assistance through a Protection and Advocacy office in your state (see Appendix A). Some private attorneys also take selected cases on a contingency fee, meaning that they get paid only if you win your appeal. Talk to your state or local bar association for referrals.

SOCIAL SECURITY SURVIVORS BENEFITS

What It Is

Social Security Survivors Benefits are monthly insurance payments to children under 18 whose parents have died. When most people think of Social Security, they think of retirement benefits, but Social Security taxes also pay into survivors' insurance for certain family members, including children.

Who Is Eligible

To be eligible for Social Security Survivors Benefits, a child must be under 18 (full-time students under 19 and older disabled children are also eligible), unmarried, and the dependent of a parent who has died. The parent in question must have worked, paid Social Security taxes, and earned enough credits to generate benefits. Because my sister didn't earn enough Social Security credits before she died, my nephew Kevin wasn't eligible for survivor's benefits; he received only AFDC and Medicaid.

A child's disability is not relevant for Social Security Survivors Benefits; only the parent's work history is. According to the Social

Security Administration, 98 percent of children are eligible for benefits if a working parent should die.[21]

What You Get

Children who qualify for Social Security Survivors Benefits receive monthly cash benefits. These benefits are based on the average lifetime earnings of the parent and on how much the parent paid into Social Security. A child can receive both SSI and Social Security if she is eligible for both.

The Application Process

How It Should Work

Apply promptly by phone or at any Social Security office since in most cases benefits will only be retroactive to the date of application. Even if you don't have all your paperwork together, apply anyway. The Social Security office should help you collect any documentation you need.

What You Need to Bring

You will need original documents or certified copies of the child's Social Security card and birth certificate, the parent's Social Security number, the parent's death certificate, and the deceased parent's W-2 forms or federal tax return (if self-employed) for the most recent year. You should also bring a checkbook or savings passbook if you want the benefits deposited directly to an account each month.

ADOPTION ASSISTANCE PROGRAM (AAP)

What It Is

AAP is a federal cash assistance program that provides monthly benefits to children whose adoption may depend on financial aid. Some states also have state-run programs for children who may not be eligible for federal adoption assistance.

Foster children are eligible for financial, social, and medical assistance, including Medicaid, all of which they typically lose when they are adopted. Most adoptive parents willingly shoulder the financial responsibility for these children in exchange for the security of adoption. With respect to some children, however, there are circumstances that place added burdens on their caregivers: They may suffer from a physical disability or an emotional disorder, or they may be part of a sibling group that must be placed together. Relatives or foster parents who care for these children may depend on the government assistance they receive; it may be that they simply cannot afford to adopt the child without it. AAP is designed to provide the financial assistance to encourage the adoption of these "special needs" children.

Adoption assistance lasts until the child is 18 years old. It can be discontinued earlier if the adoptive parent is no longer legally responsible for the support of the child, and states can extend eligibility to age 21 if the child is physically or mentally disabled.

Who Is Eligible

Special needs children are children who have situations or conditions that make it difficult to find an adoptive home for them without assistance. These might include age, race, or ethnicity; a background of severe neglect or abuse; inclusion in a sibling group; a family history of mental illness; or a disability (physical, medical, mental, or emotional). Exactly which situations and conditions create "special needs" may change from state to state. While AAP is funded by the federal government, each state defines its own eligibility requirements.

Before he can be considered a special needs child, the state must verify that a child cannot or should not be returned to his family, that he is free for adoption, and that reasonable efforts have been made to place him in a family without financial aid.

There are also financial requirements for AAP, which serves children who would have received federal assistance if they had not been adopted. Therefore, federal AAP benefits are available only to children who (1) are getting federal foster care payments at the time of adoption, (2) are receiving or are eligible to receive SSI at the time of adoption, or (3) can show AFDC eligibility at the time they were removed from their parents and at the time of adoption. As is true for AFDC, your income should not affect your grandchild's eligibility for AAP, although it will affect the amount of monthly aid he receives. A state-run AAP program may have financial qualifications that differ from those of the federal program.

What You Get

Children who are eligible receive monthly cash payments, medical assistance, and, occasionally, additional social services. Adoptive parents may also be eligible for reimbursement for one-time, or "nonrecurring," adoption expenses, which may include adoption fees, court costs, and attorney fees.

AAP cash benefits are negotiated between the administering agency and your family and are based on your financial circumstances and the particular needs of the child you are adopting. Actual rates vary from state to state, but they cannot be more than the family foster care (Youakim) benefits for which your grandchild would be eligible.

Medical assistance is available to children who have special medical needs that are already present or that may appear later on. Children who qualify for the federal program automatically receive Medicaid. Medicaid coverage varies from state to state, and some states cover children who are not federally eligible.

Some AAP agreements also include services like respite care, specialized day care, counseling, and other social services that might be provided to foster parents.

The Application Process

How It Should Work

The Adoption Assistance Agreement is a legal document that is negotiated between the adoptive parent and the state or county adoption agency. Each agreement is based on the needs of the particular child. The agreement specifies the amount of the payments; the eligibility requirements for Medicaid and social services; and the other payments, services, and assistance programs that are available. The agreement includes wording that guarantees that it will be in effect regardless of what state you live in, and it includes provisions to protect the child's interests if you move to a new state.

You can apply for adoption assistance when you begin the adoption process. Sometimes an adoption worker will deliver a proposed AAP agreement when she comes to assess your home. Otherwise, make sure you ask about it. Once you do apply, look at the initial agreement carefully. If it is not acceptable, negotiate it *before* the adoption goes through. Afterward, you must report any change in your family circumstances, and you must recertify the agreement on a regular schedule set by your state.

▪ WHAT YOU NEED TO KNOW

▪ *Adoption assistance isn't a favor.* If your grandchild qualifies for AAP, he is entitled to it. Find out what your state's criteria for AAP are, and don't be afraid to ask.

▪ *Negotiation should precede adoption.* Negotiate and sign the AAP agreement before you adopt your grandchild. Once the adoption is final, the state has no incentive to negotiate with you.

▪ *Even negotiation for AAP benefits for at-risk children should precede adoption.* Think ahead. Your grandchild may not appear to have serious problems, but certain circumstances like prenatal drug exposure or a mentally ill parent could make her vulnerable to problems in the future. According to attorney Pamela Mohr,[22] if you have reason to believe that your grandchild is at risk for future problems, some states allow you to apply for AAP; the agreement you sign will say that your grandchild does not qualify for AAP now but that her eligibility can be addressed again if problems arise in the future. However, you must negotiate this agreement and complete the paperwork before you adopt your grandchild.

▪ *It's a good idea to talk to a legal expert.* An attorney or an advocate can help you understand the various services and assistance to which your grandchild may be entitled. He can also identify which services are most important to the child, negotiate modifications of the agreement, enforce the agreement, or appeal decisions. If you have an attorney handling your adoption, talk to him about AAP. If not, consider talking to someone. I know a grandmother in Pittsburgh who adopted her grandchild. When she asked about assistance, the social worker asked her why she wasn't happy enough to get her grandchild and why she needed to apply for money, too. Sometimes it's easier to have a professional handle these issues for you.

HEALTH CARE AND NUTRITION ASSISTANCE

Any parent knows that children run up a small fortune in health care costs. They need vaccinations and school physicals. They get colds, scrapes, and a collection of childhood diseases. The more adventuresome ones sprain and break things as they test their limits and endurance. Moreover, the cost of doctors and medicine is exorbitant. If you add the health risks of prenatal drug exposure or the cost of psychiatric care for traumatized children, your health care costs can run sky-high.

Unlike parents, who can get insurance for their children, most grandparents cannot put grandchildren on their insurance policies. A few rare employers have allowed grandkids to be included when a grandparent has guardianship, but most grandparents must adopt their grandchildren in order to get private health insurance for them. This is where government benefits become very important. Even middle-class grandparents, who may be able to financially support their grandchildren, need the medical benefits that come with AFDC, SSI, and Youakim.

MEDICAID

What It Is

Medicaid is a health care program for people with low income and limited assets; it helps pay doctor and hospital bills and some medications. However, Medicaid is not so much one program as 50 individual programs, with each state providing a different combination of benefits. Although the states all function within the same federal guidelines, there is significant variety in eligibility criteria, as well as in the conditions and treatments covered. What follows is a brief and broad explanation of Medicaid benefits. This information always needs to be confirmed by someone at your state level.

Who Is Eligible

Although Medicaid varies from state to state, children who qualify for AFDC, Youakim, and SSI automatically qualify for Medicaid. Additionally, many poor children who don't qualify for financial assistance through AFDC or SSI may still be eligible for Medicaid coverage. Check with your local office to find out if your grandchild is eligible.

What You Get

Medicaid coverage can vary greatly from state to state. However, all participating states must provide children with medically necessary doctor and hospital services, lab work and X rays, and early screening. In many cases, additional medical services, like prescription drugs, eyeglasses, dental care, counseling, and inpatient psychiatric care for individuals under 21, are also provided. (See "Early Periodic Screening, Diagnosis, and Treatment," below.)

The Application Process

How It Should Work

In many states Medicaid comes automatically with AFDC, SSI, and Youakim eligibility; the forms might even come together. In other states you will have to sign up for it separately. Be sure to ask. Medicaid coverage is supposed to take effect within 45 days of your application and be retroactive to the day you applied. Additionally, states must provide Medicaid to the child for the three months before the application was filed, if he or she would have been eligible at that time.

How It Often Works

Unfortunately, processing a Medicaid application often takes much longer than 45 days, and a medically needy grandchild could exhaust your resources while you wait. Don't let it happen. If you have a problem or an emergency, call your eligibility or welfare worker.

■ WHAT YOU NEED TO KNOW

Once your grandchild's benefits begin, you will need to find doctors who accept payment through Medicaid. Because of lower reimbursement rates and the paperwork involved, many doctors are reluctant to accept it. If you run into problems, remember that most county hospitals, county clinics, and free clinics are good resources.

EARLY PERIODIC SCREENING, DIAGNOSIS, AND TREATMENT (EPSDT)

What It Is

EPSDT is a provision of the federal Medicaid program that specifically addresses the needs of children. It is designed to provide financially needy children with preventive health care by detecting and treating early signs of disease or disability and by connecting them with ongoing, comprehensive medical assistance. Federal policy defines the parameters of EPSDT programs, but they are administered by individual state programs whose names and regulations may vary. In California, for instance, EPSDT is handled through a program called Child Health and Disability Prevention (CHDP). It may have another name in your state. EPSDT is a critical program for your grandchildren because it provides many services that may not be available to adult Medicaid recipients.

Who Is Eligible

Every child who is eligible for Medicaid is eligible for federally funded EPSDT services. (See "Medicaid," above.) Some states also provide early screening and prevention services to low-income children who are not eligible for Medicaid. If your grandchildren are not eligible for Medicaid, ask state resources if there is a state-funded program that applies to them.

What You Get

Services include free childhood screening and free medically necessary follow-up diagnosis and treatment for conditions found during the EPSDT screens.

Screening

Regular well-baby and well-child checkups are the foundation of the EPSDT program. These typically include a full unclothed physical exam; assessment of physical and mental health development; vision, hearing, and dental screening; health education; a nutrition check; age-appropriate vaccinations and booster shots; and appropriate or necessary lab tests, including tests for lead poisoning. However, states vary in how well they carry out these requirements.

Diagnosis and Treatment

Your grandchild is entitled to a broad range of free diagnosis and treatment services through EPSDT. Your state should provide "medically necessary" corrective treatment for any physical or mental illness or condition that is suspected or detected during an EPSDT screen, as long as it is covered by federal Medicaid. This means that EPSDT may require your state to provide certain services to children even though it may not provide those same services to adult Medicaid recipients. These services can include assessment for and provision of glasses, hearing aids, and medical equipment; dental care to relieve pain and infection; dental health maintenance and teeth restoration; rehabilitation; respiratory care; home health services; and inpatient or outpatient services to evaluate physical or mental illness.

Although each state may have its own definition for "medically necessary," federal law requires every state to provide diagnostic and treatment services "to correct or ameliorate defects and physical and mental illnesses and conditions discovered by the screening services."[23]

Additional Help and Information

State agencies are obligated to inform the caregivers of all eligible children about EPSDT and to make those services available to them. To this end, you should be provided with a list of specific EPSDT providers near you, as well as their addresses. You should also be offered scheduling and transportation assistance, if you need it, for your grandchildren's regularly scheduled checkups.

The Application Process

How It Should Work

You should be offered information on EPSDT services when you apply for AFDC, Youakim, SSI, or Medicaid for your grandchildren. If your grandchild is eligible (and most GAP grandchildren should be), you can schedule an appointment through whichever state or county agency administers the program.

Your grandchild's periodic checkups should be scheduled on a regular basis determined by your state. However, you are entitled to request additional screens whenever these are needed to determine the existence of a new disease or condition or whenever an existing condition seems to change or worsen. For instance, if your granddaughter starts to squint in school, you may request a vision screening even if her next scheduled appointment is several months away.

How It Often Works

Grandparents are rarely informed about EPSDT services, and while federal guidelines require states to use broader standards when providing services to children, many states still apply the stricter adult Medicaid standards. Thus, states frequently deny services to children even though the services are covered by EPSDT.[24]

▪ WHAT YOU NEED TO KNOW

▪ *EPSDT is an important resource for your grandchildren.* If it is offered to you, take it. If it is not offered, ask for it. Many people turn down these services because they think they are unnecessary if they have Medicaid. Whereas Medicaid is designed to treat illness, EPSDT is designed for early detection and prevention. Without early intervention, many conditions, including mental health problems and learning disabilities, can become more difficult and costly to treat.

▪ *Not all Medicaid providers handle EPSDT services.* Make sure you get a specific list of those who do.

▪ *Many providers are poorly informed.* There are a number of private EPSDT providers and personnel in county facilities who are not aware of the full extent of early screening and treatment benefits. They may not be aware that additional (interperiodic) screens and checkups are allowed, or they may be reluctant to provide them because reimbursement is slow. They may also mistakenly bill you for services that should be paid for by the state. If this happens, photocopy the bill and send it back to the doctor with a letter of explanation. Always keep a copy for yourself.

▪ *Many states don't fully implement federal EPSDT regulations.* As with many government programs, there can be a discrepancy between federal EPSDT ideals and state practice. For instance, while mental health assessment and dental care follow-ups are both required by federal law, some state programs may not offer them. If you have problems receiving EPSDT services for your grandchild, you can ask for a hearing. Contact your local Legal Aid or Protection and Advocacy chapters for help (see Appendix A).

FOOD STAMPS

What It Is

Food stamps are checks or coupons that can be used in the grocery store like money. You can use food stamps to buy food or seeds to grow food. You cannot use them to purchase items like diapers, toilet paper, tobacco, alcohol, or pet food.

Who Is Eligible

Many families who receive AFDC are entitled to food stamps. However, your grandchild's eligibility for food stamps, unlike AFDC, will be affected by your income and the income of everyone in your household. For purposes of food stamp eligibility, a household is a family or group of individuals who live in the same place and prepare food together. If you and your grandchild are *both* receiving AFDC, it is likely that you are both entitled to food stamps. However, if your grandchild is getting AFDC and you are not, he may not be eligible because your income would be counted on his application.

What You Get

The amount of food stamps you can receive depends on a number of factors, including your income, your resources, how many people are in your household, and the cost of your living expenses. Your eligibility worker should be able to tell you which resources can be counted against your eligibility.

The Application Process

How It Should Work

You can apply for food stamps through your state or local welfare office at the same time you apply for AFDC. In some states the application form for food stamps comes as part of the same application package.

▪ WHAT YOU NEED TO KNOW

▪ *It always pays to apply.* Many grandparents either are too embarrassed to apply for food stamps or believe they won't qualify. If there is any possibility that you and your grandchildren may be eligible for food stamps, apply for them. Raising children is an expensive proposition; you deserve any help you can get.

▪ *You have a right to a "fair hearing."* Request one if you do not qualify for food stamps, and you feel you were unfairly denied or if you need to address mistakes or unfair treatment.

▪ *Keeping records is necessary.* If you do qualify, keep receipts and bills for all your purchases. You will have to report changes in your income and expenses on a regular basis, and you may need receipts to verify your records.

SPECIAL SUPPLEMENTAL FOOD PROGRAM FOR WOMEN, INFANTS AND CHILDREN (WIC)

What It Is

WIC is a nutrition education and supplemental food program for low-income mothers, infants, and children who are at health risk. WIC originates in the U.S. Department of Agriculture and is administered by either a health or human services agency in each state.

Who Is Eligible

Low-income mothers, infants, and children who are at health risk are eligible for WIC. It can continue from birth to two to five years of age, depending on the state. Although grandparents are not eligible for these benefits, grandchildren may qualify. Eligibility is determined by your income and the health needs of the child (a drug-exposed infant, for instance, is definitely at a health risk).

What You Get

WIC is similar to food stamps in that you get checks or vouchers to be used at the grocery store like money. However, WIC vouchers are earmarked for specific foods that support the nutritional needs of the child. For instance, one voucher may be for a dozen eggs, another for a quart of milk or for infant formula. Those who are eligible also receive educational information about nutrition and child development through a class or a counselor. Finally, you can use WIC as a referral center for other appropriate health care services for your grandchild.

The Application Process

How It Should Work

You can start your application for WIC by calling your county health department or your state social services or welfare office. If they don't handle the WIC program in your area, they can refer you to the agency that does. Once you call, a WIC worker may be able to do a preliminary screening by phone, asking you questions about your income. If you meet these first requirements, the worker will schedule an interview for you and your grandchild.

Three things happen in the interview at the clinic or office. First, you are given a second, more in-depth, screening for income. If you meet this requirement, your grandchild will be screened for "health risk" criteria: An assessment of her diet is made on the basis of what the child ate in the last 24 hours, she is tested for anemia by means of a finger-stick blood test and is weighed and measured, and a health questionnaire on the child is filled out. This package determines whether the child is eligible.

WIC determines eligibility on the spot; you won't have to wait days to find out. In most states you get your first vouchers before you leave the office. However, as with all benefits, delivery varies from state to state. Once you qualify for WIC, you are certified for six months. You will then be recertified every six months until the child is no longer eligible.

How It Often Works

Applying for WIC vouchers involves another appointment, another meeting, another place to haul your grandchild, and more forms to fill out. None of this is made easy for you. Moreover, because WIC is not fully funded, not every child who is technically eligible gets covered. When states cut back, they do so by age, dropping the upper age limit from five years to four or three or even younger.

▪ WHAT YOU NEED TO KNOW

If you have a child under the age of five, apply for this! Many grandparents hear about the income qualification and assume they won't qualify. Since WIC allows income levels higher than AFDC, Medicaid, or food stamps, you may still meet the WIC criteria even if you have a retirement income.[25] Even if your grandchild doesn't qualify for this program, WIC can be a good first line of referral to other health care services.

WHERE TO LOOK FOR ADDITIONAL SERVICES IN YOUR STATE

This chapter has only reviewed basic federal assistance that may be available to your grandchildren. You might also look into government-funded Head Start programs as a source of day care as well as early childhood education and socialization for very young grandchildren.

Many states and communities have independent programs and organizations that support children and families in need. Survivors of crime victims can often receive financial assistance for funerals or counseling through programs developed to assist this population. State or local public health offices and community health centers may provide free or low-cost health care for children. Religious and charitable organizations like Catholic Charities, Jewish Family Services, and Family Service America may offer help with food, clothing, and transportation. Churches, synagogues, and community centers may sponsor child care and after-school activities, as well as camp scholarships for fixed-income children.

Ask your grandchild's teacher or doctor about additional local resources. Find out if your area has an information and referral line. And don't forget grandparent support groups. In addition to providing emotional support, some grandparent groups help with general assistance, and they are a wonderful source of information.

CHAPTER 13 | Special Education
and Early Intervention

> If you've told a child a thousand times and he
> still does not understand, then it is not the child
> who is a slow learner.
> —*Walter Barbee*[1]

E ver since 1954, when the U.S. Supreme Court
ruled to desegregate schools in *Brown v.
Board of Education*, American children have
enjoyed the right to equal education.[2] But if your grandchild cannot
see the blackboard, read the alphabet, remember instructions, or
stay in her seat, she cannot take advantage of the education she is
entitled to, no matter how good that education may be.

Fortunately, the civil rights movement of the 1960s also drew
attention to the rights of the handicapped, including the need of
disabled children for equal access to their equal education. Congress
therefore passed laws that gave states a financial incentive to offer
special resources to kids with disabilities.[3]

Children having serious difficulties in school are entitled to a
number of special education programs and services to help them
make the most of their public education. Two particular federal laws,
or parts of them, apply to children with special education needs:

Section 504 of the Rehabilitation Act of 1973 prohibits discrimination against the disabled in any program that receives federal
funds, including schools.[4] If your grandchild has a disability
that limits certain activities but does not affect his academic

performance, he may be entitled to modifications in the class-room and curriculum through Section 504.

IDEA (Individuals with Disabilities Education Act, formerly Public Law 94-142) requires all states and territories to provide a "free appropriate public education" (FAPE) to all children with disabilities and defines the rights of those children and their parents or guardians.[5] "Appropriate" means that the curriculum meets the special education needs of each child's disability. If your grandchild's disabilities seriously hinder his academic achievement, he may be eligible for special education services through IDEA.

A "free appropriate public education" is a right and an entitlement, not a privilege. It is implemented through a procedure called an IEP, or Individualized Education Program. This is a detailed plan of special services, tailored to the needs of each child, which the school must provide to ensure that the child's education is indeed "appropriate."

The IEP is considered the centerpiece of special education law, and each stage of the special education process is a stepping stone toward completing it: the assessment of the child through a battery of tests, observations, and reports; meetings of teachers, professionals, and parents (or, in this case, grandparents) to evaluate whether the child qualifies for services and which services would help him; and the IEP itself, which must be carried out by the school or school district.

This process helps determine whether the problems a child is exhibiting are due to a physical, emotional, or learning disability and suggests how an environment might be created that would enable him to benefit from his public school education. This can mean individual tutoring, putting the child in a special class in the current school, or transferring to another school, whether public or private, that can better handle the disability.

"Free appropriate public education. Those are the buzz words," warns attorney Larry Hanna, special education commissioner for the Los Angeles Unified School District. "You get a compact VW, not a Rolls Royce or a Mercedes. You don't get services that are going to make you an Einstein; you get the services that will get you through, give you an even playing field." Even so, an even playing field can mean the difference between getting an education and slipping through the cracks for a child with ADHD or a learning disability.

According to the U.S. Department of Education, approximately five percent of all school children get special education services. However, nearly one-fourth of them eventually drop out.[7] The more you can learn about the special education process and the IEP, the better you can use it as a tool to provide your grandchild with an education that will allow him to learn.

THE SPECIAL EDUCATION PROCESS

The Request

The special education process begins with a written request to your local school. Anyone—a teacher, a therapist, a pediatrician, a parent or guardian, or, in your case, a grandparent—can request a special education evaluation for a child. No matter how small your town is, the school should know about the IEP. Your grandchild may have to go to another school or district for the evaluation—some areas have created a consortium among several schools to handle this—but you must still start the process with a written request to your local school. Date the letter and keep a copy for your files. This request will start a clock ticking; the school district is required to process eligibility for special education within a prescribed time frame. That time frame is dictated by state law, and many school districts fall behind their prescribed schedules. (The schedule in this chapter represents *California* law. Your own state's time frame may be different, so find out what it is. Don't let the school drag the process out so that your grandchild falls further behind.)

The Evaluation or Assessment Plan

Once the school receives your request, it has *15 days* (in California) to send you a plan for how it will evaluate your grandchild. This is a key step; don't take it lightly. The kind of testing done in the assessment will determine the kinds of services your grandchild is eligible to receive. If the child needs psychological counseling or speech therapy but those tests are not included in the assessment plan, they won't be considered in the IEP.

What testing do you want the school to do? If you don't know, take the plan to someone who can help you. You need to make sure the school is offering the right assessment for this child at this age and with these particular needs. Assessments are expensive; with budgets tight, school districts do try to cut corners where they can. You have to be the child's best advocate. Persistence and perseverance do pay off. If the assessment plan is adequate, sign and return it. If not, write in the additional tests you want before you send it back.

The Actual Assessment or Evaluation

Once you return the signed plan, the school district has *50 calendar days* (in California) to complete the assessment, which is a multidisciplinary evaluation usually conducted by a school psychologist, educational diagnostician, social worker, and other evaluators. This evaluation includes medical, educational, psychological, and sociological components. Try to get as much input into this process as possible. If you think the school's assessment is inadequate, and if you can afford it, you can have your own assessment done privately. If the final IEP reflects issues raised in your assessment, but not in the school's, the district may have to repay your costs.[8]

The Eligibility Meeting

Once the assessment is complete, the school district will schedule a meeting to determine if the child is eligible for special education services. However, some state and local agencies combine the eligibility meeting and the IEP meeting (see below) into a single conference.

What Determines Eligibility?

According to federal regulations, all "children with disabilities" are eligible for special education and related services. This includes children who have been evaluated as being mentally retarded, physically handicapped, health-impaired, or seriously emotionally disturbed, or as having specific learning disabilities. However, terms like "emotionally disturbed" and "learning disabled" are hard to define, and the final criteria for special education eligibility varies from state to state.

You might think your grandchild is learning disabled—and by many standards she may be—but the child must fit your state's criteria to be eligible for services. For instance, if your state defines a learning disabled child as one of normal intelligence who is two years behind her age-group but your dyslexic granddaughter is only one year behind, she may not qualify for special education in that state.

Even if your grandchild is not eligible for an IEP through the Individuals with Disabilities Evaluation Act, she should be able to get certain classroom modifications through Section 504. These might include having your grandchild placed at the front of the classroom, allowing her to use a tape recorder in class, or giving her more time to complete certain tests and assignments.

If it is determined that your grandchild does have a disability that makes her eligible for an IEP, the school district or public agency has up to 30 days to hold an IEP meeting.

The IEP Meeting

The IEP meeting itself can take place in any number of places—a district office, a hospital, your home—but it is most commonly held in your grandchild's own school. It should be held at a time and place that is mutually agreeable to school personnel and you, as the child's guardian.

The IEP is based on a team concept: A group of professionals work with the parents (or grandparents) and, if appropriate, the child to determine what services his special education will include. The team players are the school administrator or principal, the child's teacher, the school nurse, and a psychologist.

During the IEP meeting this team will examine your grandchild's test results, profiles, class work, teacher reports, nurse's reports, and any other material that is presented as pertinent. If a psychologist or a doctor needs to present information in person, this is where it happens. If a medical doctor is scheduled to be present, try to have your grandchild's own doctor there as well. Remember, you are an important part of this team. As primary caregiver, you are the one who knows your grandchild best, and no services can be provided without your consent.

Several things are decided at the IEP meeting: goals and objectives, placement, related services, and, for some children, transition services. The IEP form will be filled out on the basis of these decisions, and the IEP will become the blueprint or game plan for your grandchild's education.

Goals and Objectives

If your grandchild is found eligible for special education services, the next thing to decide is what kind of program and services are needed. What are your grandchild's specific disabilities? What does he need to learn to catch up to other children his age? These are the questions that must be addressed at the IEP meeting. These questions should be answered with specific goals and objectives and a schedule for measuring whether or not they are being achieved. For instance, if Carrie is a bright fifth grader who tests at a second grade reading level, she clearly needs help with reading comprehension. But her IEP should say more than "Carrie will get help with reading." Instead, Carrie's IEP goals might state that "Carrie will be able to read at a third grade level by the end of the first semester. By the end of the year, Carrie will be reading on a fourth grade level." The goals should also state which test will measure this progress.

Goals and objectives are critical in deciding which kind of placement and services your grandchild is eligible for in the coming year. Make sure they can be measured objectively. A teacher's observation or opinion is not an objective measurement.

Placement

The law requires that each child be placed in the "least restrictive environment." That means having the child in as much of a regular school program as possible while accommodating his special needs. Special options can range from extra help in a mainstream class to residential placement. Other possibilities include special day classes, a resource specialist for tutoring, state school, or, occasionally, a private school paid for by the school district. If your grandchild does need a special school and there are none in your area, he may be sent out of the district.

Related Services

If a child qualifies for special education, school districts are also supposed to provide certain additional services to help her come up to speed. "Related services" can include speech and language services, psychological counseling, special readers, tutoring, medical services in school, parent training, physical and occupational therapy, adaptive physical education, and even transportation if you live far from a special education program.

Transition Services

The IEP is designed not only to help disabled children graduate but to help older children with disabilities make the transition to life after school. Thus, an IEP could include not only special instruction but employment or college counseling, certain community experiences, and even instruction in specific daily living skills like filling out applications, handling money, and finding living arrangements. Starting at no later than 16 years old (and sometimes at 14 or younger) your grandchild's IEP should include a plan for the transition services he will need to move on in life.

Remember, although the IEP works on a team concept, it is also a negotiation session. Your concern is your grandchild's needs, but the school must focus on hundreds of children and must do so with dwindling funds. Since it is expensive to put kids in special classes and nonpublic schools, a school district does resist. "The school district is battling the budget," says education commissioner Hanna. "So the less they give you, the more they have and the happier they are."[9] On the other hand, the more prepared you are, the more you can get out of the system.

The IEP

The product of the IEP process is the actual IEP, the written Individual Education Program that you as the child's guardian must approve and sign before services can take effect. Read the IEP carefully before you sign it. Make sure it does what it is meant to do. Ask yourself the following questions:

> Is it comprehensive? A good IEP should cover every area of your grandchild's development, including behavior, socialization, communication, self-help, academic, and motor skills.

Is it specific? Are goals and objectives clearly stated in terms of objective, observable, and measurable behavior?

Is it sequential? Does it offer a solid step-by-step plan to teach your grandchild what she needs to learn?

Is it realistic and appropriate? Does it match your grandchild's current abilities? Does it encourage growth at a reasonable rate?

Is it understandable? Is it written in language that you can comfortably follow and discuss?

Was it mutually developed? In other words, were you an active part of the IEP team and does the final plan reflect your concerns?

Is it designed to close the gap between the child's ability and her achievement?

Remember, the IEP is key to your grandchild's education; you want to make sure the door it opens is the right one.

Don't Do This Yourself

Even the most sophisticated, resourceful grandparent can find the IEP process to be overwhelming. You have to tell strangers how badly off your grandchild is, and that can be hard to do without getting emotionally involved. The forms can be confusing, and the process can drag on until you run out of patience. It is good to learn the terminology and the process, but you have enough to do already without having to learn all the detailed procedures of educational law and the difference between various types of assessment plans.

The individual who helps you negotiate an IEP with your grandchild's school could be an attorney or advocate, a therapist or social worker, even another grandparent or a friend. A local education attorney or advocate knows the ropes: whom to ask, what to ask, and what to ask for. She may have even worked with this IEP team before. An educational therapist, a psychologist, or a social worker can evaluate the assessment plan and help fill out the IEP form with your wish list. These professionals have a better grasp of what are reasonable goals for your grandchild at his age and with his particular psychological and educational background. If you can't find or afford an advocate, look for another grandparent or parent who has been through this before; ask that parent to go to the IEP meeting with you. At the very least, take a friend or relative for support. Despite what anyone may tell you, you do have the right to have someone there.

Preparing for the IEP Meeting

The more information you have before your first IEP, the fewer problems you are likely to encounter. Here are some things you can do to prepare yourself for the IEP meeting:

▪ *Learn about your and your grandchild's rights.* Your grandchild has rights and so do you, as the primary caregiver or guardian. Get copies of federal rules and regulations (IDEA and Section 504), your state rules and regulations for special education, and the policies in effect in your school district. Remember, the only interpretation that ultimately counts is the federal one.

▪ *Find out the chain of command in your school district.* If you are not satisfied with the outcome of the IEP meeting and need to go higher up, you will already know whom to go to.

▪ *Keep records.* Write down the names and numbers of everyone you talk to. They could be helpful later on.

▪ *Review your grandchild's school records.* Go to the school and photocopy everything that is in the child's cumulative and confidential reports. You may have to check in different departments to get all of them. If the child has ever been in any kind of facility, get their records as well. Copy everything: handwritten notes, notes scribbled on the folder or jacket, any work the child has done. You are arming yourself on all fronts.

▪ *Speak with the psychologist.* Find out who the psychologist is and get her reports on your grandchild. Be nice about this; presume that the psychologist is doing the best job she can for the child. If you are using an advocate, he will know how to ask the right questions.

▪ *Request your own copy of the assessment report.*

▪ *If you have had an outside assessment done, plan to bring it.* Or, if possible, bring along the expert who did the assessment; he or she may be able to provide additional information.

▪ *Gather outside information.* Collect medical records and any school or test records the school district may not have. Because reports don't tell you everything about a child, be sure to bring in real-life examples of your grandchild's abilities and disabilities in different areas. Talk to other adults who come into contact with your grandchild—doctors, social workers, clergy members, even family and neighbors. Ask them to put their comments and observations in writing. Submit this information for the assessment.

▪ *Set your own goals for your grandchild.* If you let the school district define all of your grandchild's goals and objectives, it may only offer minimal services and will probably not address all your grandchild's needs. Make a list of what things your grandchild can do and what you think he should learn during the school year. Get blank copies of the IEP forms, photocopy them, and fill them in. Focus on your goals for your grandchild and how you want them to be accomplished. Does he have problems hopping or jumping? Ask for adaptive physical education. This is your wish list.

▪ *Think about placement.* What do you want for your grandchild? Talk to someone who knows your school district and ask the following questions: What special classrooms are available? What do they offer? Where are there special schools? Inspect any classroom or school where you think they might place your grandchild. Interview the teacher. If you're not happy with the placement, take in your own plan. You may have a fight on your hands, but it could be worth it. You might even be able to get your grandchild placed in a private school, but that is a difficult proposition.

▪ *Ask for therapy.* One important goal that is often overlooked is psychological counseling. Being in a special education classroom, as helpful as it is, has a stigma that is hard on children. Their self-esteem is low. Other children may tease. Always try to get mental health testing and psychological counseling into your grandchild's IEP, and make sure that it is with a trained therapist. The school may view sessions with a guidance counselor as therapy, but many guidance counselors may not be qualified to deal with the issues your grandchild may be experiencing.

▪ *Consider nonacademic activities.* Lunch, recess, physical education, and activities like art and music are important parts of the school day. Make sure your grandchild's IEP lets her take advantage of the nonacademic part of school as well.

▪ *Carefully consider having your grandchild at the meeting.* Despite what anyone may tell you, you are entitled to have the child present. The question is, Do you want to? The IEP process can be devastating. Personally, I don't recommend that a young child be present at an IEP meeting. Perhaps a high school student may be confident enough to provide some input, but I can't think of a good reason to have an elementary school child present. These children have such fragile self-esteem that they can't help but be affected by everyone talking about their problems. However, your grandchild must eventually learn to become his own advocate.

▪ *Be vigilant.* In so many arenas you have had to step gingerly with bureacracy; this is one place you must be willing to push. Just because public schools have a duty to identify children who need special education doesn't mean they always do so. Children get lost in the school system. The ones who are quiet and nice may get Cs or Ds and yet be passed along without services. One little girl was denied special education services because the school blamed her problems on her "dysfunctional family" (she lived with her grandparents). Only after a long legal fight did her grandfather manage to place her in a residential program for the learning disabled.[10]

Don't back down. "The people I see who are the noisiest, who go down to the schools and bug them, they're the ones who get the services they need," says Hanna.[11] So, even if you have an advocate, be vigilant.

During the IEP Meeting

▪ *Be confident.* Your image may affect how school personnel respond to you. Bring your own set of rules, regulations, and supporting material. Have your grandchild's file organized neatly and in chronological order; keep state and federal regulations in a separate folder. This way you also look prepared. Speak clearly and maintain eye contact. And remember, this committee is paid to work *for* you and your grandchild; they are not dispensing favors. Special education is a right, not a privilege.

▪ *Have people sign in.* Pass around a sign-in sheet at the beginning of the meeting. This will let you address everyone by name.

▪ *Ask questions.* Especially when you don't understand something, ask about it. You have a right to simple explanations of anything that is unclear to you.

▪ *Repeat what you are asking for.* Do this as often as necessary. To quote the Coordinating Council for Handicapped Children: "You are not at the IEP to discuss the limitations of the school budget. You are there to determine what your child needs to have an appropriate education."[12]

▪ *If necessary, request another meeting.* If you cannot come to an agreement, are running out of time or need more time to think, you have the right to request another meeting. You do not have to make a decision at that moment.

▪ *Don't sign the IEP until you understand and accept it.* Remember, you do not have to sign an unsatisfactory IEP. If you do not agree with the school's evaluation, you can get an independent evaluation and request a new meeting based on it. You can also file an appeal through a mediation process or a "due process hearing" (see below).

After the IEP Meeting

▪ *Request your own copy of the final IEP.*

▪ *Follow your grandchild's progress closely.* Periodically ask the teachers for a progress report. Remember, you can initiate changes or a review if your grandchild is not improving. You can also request another IEP meeting.

▪ *Ask teachers what you can do at home to help.* Many skills your grandchild will be learning at school can be practiced at home.

▪ *Keep records.* Record all questions and comments you want to discuss with the school, meetings and phone conversations you want to remember, and any information that may be useful in future reviews and evaluations. It is easy to forget what you don't write down.

▪ *Try to resolve any problems you have with the school within the school district.* On the other hand, if you cannot come to an agreement with school officials and your grandchild is not being properly supported, you can file an appeal.

The Appeal Process

If the final IEP is not acceptable to you and you cannot resolve the issue with the school district, you can appeal. Some states offer a mediation process first, but any issues that cannot be resolved in mediation will be taken to a due process hearing. Likewise, if the

IEP is not being followed, you can file a formal complaint with your state board of education, the U.S. Department of Education, or the Office of Civil Rights and start an investigation. You are entitled to be present when your complaint comes before the board of education. Sometimes, if the school district thinks you will fight them all the way to a hearing, they may give you what you want—it's cheaper. If the due process hearing is not satisfactory, the appeal process can go on to a U.S. district court and, in some cases, up to the U.S. Supreme Court.

If you do start the appeal process, you may want to consult an attorney or advocate. Most states have Protection and Advocacy agencies that can provide you with guidance. So look around before you decide you can't afford representation. And don't be afraid to "rock the boat." A free *appropriate* public education is a right that belongs to your grandchild; you have a right to make sure that what is provided is appropriate.

The Review Process

Once your grandchild has started the IEP process, she will be reviewed annually and reassessed at a minimum of every three years to see if her needs are being met and progress is being made and to determine what changes are needed as the child gets older. The IEP may also be revised anytime you see a need for revision and make a request.

EARLY INTERVENTION AND SPECIAL EDUCATION SERVICES FOR INFANTS, TODDLERS, AND PRESCHOOLERS WITH DISABILITIES

One of the wonderful things about IDEA is the possibility of early intervention, that is, of addressing the needs of disabled children before they enter the school system and start to fall behind. Federal law extends special education assistance to preschool children as young as three years, and, in some states, to infants and toddlers (birth to two years).[13] Children who are at risk for developing disabilities, such as drug-exposed infants, are also eligible in a number of places.

The goal of early intervention is to identify and treat problems and delays in children as soon as possible. This can be as simple as prescribing glasses for a three-year-old or as intensive as complete physical therapy for an infant with cerebral palsy. The theory is that the more special assistance a child receives early on, when the rate of learning is fastest, the fewer the special education services he may need later in life.

The process of applying for early intervention is similar to applying for the IEP and involves the following stages:

The Request

Make a request, in writing, for an evaluation and assessment of your grandchild's eligibility and needs. Start the process at your local school, just as you would if the child were already enrolled there; speak to the principal or someone in charge of special education. If you have any problems, call your state's department of education and ask who in your area is responsible for special education programs for preschoolers with disabilities. If your grandchild is under three, ask about early intervention services for infants and toddlers; they are not offered in every state.

The Assessment

Your grandchild will be evaluated by a team of professionals, which may include a psychologist and an occupational or a physical therapist as well as other experts, depending on the rules and regulations of your state. You are an important part of this team and should participate as much as you can in this process. Many of the preparation suggestions for the IEP apply here (see above).

The Plan

If your grandchild is eligible for special education programs or early intervention, the assessment team will create an IFSP (Individualized Family Service Plan). Like the IEP, this plan describes the child's developmental level, the goals to be achieved, which services the child will receive, where and when she will receive these services, and what steps will be taken to ease the child's transition into school or another program.

Unlike the IEP, which focuses on the individual student, the IFSP addresses the whole family. The philosophy is that the best way to meet the needs of a small child is to work with the family. This can include family counseling, respite care, and educational services to help everyone understand and cope with your grandchild's disability.

The Services

The special education programs developed for preschoolers are free programs in public schools and are specifically designed to help children with disabilities. Early intervention services may be offered through public or private agencies in a variety of settings: clinics, hospitals, neighborhood day-care centers, the local health department, even your home. Although there is no cost for evaluation and assessment, not all early intervention services are free. However, some services may be covered under Medicaid.

Again, each state develops its own policies for carrying out the IDEA. You will need to find out about the specific policies in your state. The National Information Center for Children and Youth with Disabilities (NICHCY) publishes free resource sheets listing agencies and contact people in each state (see Appendix A for more information).

AND IT'S ANOTHER NOTEBOOK!

Lots of paperwork is generated with special needs children: assessment reports, IFSPs, IEPs, medical forms, phone numbers, conferences, growth milestones, immunizations, therapy reports, and so on. The more organized you are, the better you can protect your grandchild's right to a free and equal education.

What to Keep in Your Child's Home File

- A copy of IDEA (formerly Public Law 94-142) and its regulations.

- A copy of your state's rules and regulations on special education.
- A copy of the school's IEP procedures.
- A "chain of command" list. Keep a list or chart of the chain of command within the school system, beginning at the local level and ending with state and federal agencies. Include addresses and telephone numbers for easy reference.
- A list of school and IEP players. Every year, list your grandchild's teacher, school, principal, and psychologist, as well as any related services personnel, special education teachers, the school district superintendent, school board members, and the special education administrator.
- Copies of all school records. These may come from the child's cumulative records, psychological reports, and any other papers the school district might have about your grandchild. Keep them chronologically, with the most recent year on top.
- Report cards.
- Copies of test results and recommendations from independent assessments.
- All written (including handwritten) letters and notes to and from school personnel.
- All written communication with outside professionals regarding your grandchild's unique needs.
- Dated notes on parent–teacher conferences.
- Dated notes you have taken during conversations with the child's physician and other professionals who see your grandchild.
- Dated notes on all telephone conversations with school personnel or others regarding your grandchild.
- A list of any medications being given to your grandchild at home and at school as authorized by the child's physician. Include the kind of medicine and dosage information. In addition, note prescription numbers and any changes in dosage or reactions.

ADDITIONAL RESOURCES

There are many kinds of support and information services out there for families with disabled children, from public agencies to support groups for families of children with disabilities. Also, many states have published manuals that explain their special education and related services for children with disabilities. Contact your state Department of Education or any of the groups or organizations listed in Appendix A for more information.

ONE LAST WORD: AIM HIGH

A disability does not have to be a sentence to failure. It's not that these children can't learn—many are very smart—but they need to learn differently. Give them goals and aim high. The IEP offers transition services for adjusting to life after high school, and Section 504 of the Rehabilitation Act of 1973 prohibits discrimination against disabled applicants or students at schools that receive federal funds. There is financial aid and special programming even at many top colleges and universities. Taped textbooks, extended time for testing, tape recorders, computers, and interpreters for students with hearing problems are just a few of the modifications that are helping disabled teenagers participate and succeed on American campuses.

"Go for doctor, lawyer, not secretary," says special education commissioner Hanna, who is himself dyslexic. "The [school] will want to put them into bricklaying, truck driving. Don't let it happen."[14]

SECTION III

Strength in Numbers

CHAPTER 14 | Their Arms about Us:
Finding and Forming
Support Groups

"GAP is a place where I can go as a grandmother and let my hair down and scream and holler and say what I feel. It is a shoulder to cry on."

"GAP is a place you come to when you reach the end of your rope. Three years in court keeps you from talking about things, and you need to vent. This was the first place we were allowed to sit and cry and tell our story."

"It doesn't matter here whether you're poor or rich, black or white. We become a family here. They have become my family."

"There is no place like this. I lived in constant fear of snapping. I come here and all these mothers start picking me up and, next thing you know, I'm whole again."

"I came in here and I was a beat person. I was a rug. I'm not a rug anymore. I'm a strong person now because of GAP. I'm a human being."

"Instead of aging, I've become younger. I don't look younger, but inside I feel like a very young person. I can cope with anything now—and I am."

There are many reasons why I urge grandparents to seek out support groups, as I have repeatedly done throughout this book. Each of these reasons comes back to the same root: While you are sacrificing

243

everything to help your grandchildren, you need someone to help you. A GAP group lets you look out for one another.

A group is a fallout shelter, a place for people to come together when everything seems to be raining down on their heads and exploding around them. It is the best antidote to the overwhelming feelings of loneliness. It cuts isolation. You can cry and yell in a group and not be judged. You can make friends who understand you because they have been there. You can go to a meeting and sit next to a another grandfather who is angry at a son who won't parent or another grandmother who is frustrated with her granddaughter for disrupting her life. You can unload your concerns without criticism. It lets you see how normal your feelings are.

A group is a living library. You can find guidance from the experiences other people have had in similar situations. Someone who has already raised a grandchild to age 15 can give you specific feedback on your five-year-old. This is also a source for practical information, like phone numbers of attorneys and helpful social workers, and for assistance in navigating issues like obtaining custody or AFDC and Medicaid for the kids.

A group can also be a kind of way station, a place where basic needs can be gratified through, for example, a clothing exchange, a ride to a doctor's appointment, a new friend who might watch the kids for an hour. One support group in Las Vegas organized themselves to pay for medical exams and eyeglasses for disadvantaged grandparents. "We're not doing for the child," said its executive director. "We are doing for the grandparents so they can do for the child."[1]

FINDING A GROUP IN YOUR AREA

At last count there were over 400 grandparent groups already running in the United States.[2] Some of them are chapters or offshoots of larger organizations like Grandparents As Parents (GAP), Grandparents Raising Grandchildren, and Grandparents United for Children's Rights. Others are local, organized by individual grandparents, social workers, therapists, nurses, and even teachers. A number of support groups offer additional services, including dispensing of newsletters, resource directories, and how-to manuals; hotlines; and emergency assistance with basic needs like food, housing, and financial assistance. And many are active in political and legislative advocacy.

Appendix A is a small directory of resources; some may be able to point you to a group in your area. You should also call your local child guidance clinic or family service agency to see if the staff knows of any grandparent groups that are just starting up. If not, you may be able to convince them of the need to start one or to help you organize one.

STARTING YOUR OWN GAP GROUP

Before Your First Meeting

There are many kinds of grandparent groups across the country. Some focus on emotional support, some on basic needs and political action, and some on a combination of the three. Some of these groups are run by grandparents, others by social workers and therapists. Each, however, has had to resolve some of the same issues to get up and running.

Getting the Word Out

The first step is identifying your target population and letting them know about your group. Although GAP stands for "Grandparents As Parents," our membership extends beyond grandparents who are actually raising their grandchildren. We take grandparents who are fighting for visitation as well as grandparents whose grandchildren were returned to their parents by the system. We have even had a great aunt and a big sister show up at a meeting. I don't believe in turning away anyone who can benefit from the information and support GAP offers.

Once you get the ball rolling to start a GAP group, talk it up. Word of mouth does wonders. You never know who might know another grandparent raising a grandchild, and people strike up conversations all the time in the market, the bank, a doctor's office. In fact, most of our grandparents have GAP business cards. If they see a grandparent with a grandchild in a store, at a school meeting, or even on the street, they pass them out. There are also formal ways to spread the word:

▪ *Use your community.* You may not know other grandparents in your situation, but there are people who do. Contact local pediatricians, hospitals, social workers, attorneys, schools, churches, and synagogues. Tell them your plans and ask them to give your name and number to any grandparents they know. They cannot give you a grandparent's name—that's confidential—but they can give out your name or even send out a prepared letter. Their offices are also good places to post flyers, if you get permission first.

▪ *Use the media.* Not only are your local newspaper and radio and television stations a source of local news, they are your link to other isolated grandparents. There are two ways to get the word out through the media: meeting announcements and articles.

Most newspapers and radio stations have calendar listings of upcoming events. This is a simple way to spread the word. One group sent news releases to as many papers as possible, then followed up with a phone call to confirm. If you do this, be sure to include your name and contact number on your release.

A more challenging, but more effective, approach is the human interest story. Reporters are always on the lookout for personal stories that tie into a social trend. Contact a local newspaper and ask if they would like to do a story on your family. Make sure the article states that you are interested in starting a group for grandparents and includes a contact number. Do the same thing with local radio and television stations. When Peggy Plante wanted to start a GAP group in Quincy, Massachussetts, she called the *Patriot Ledger*. The paper ran a feature story on Plante and her GAP partner, Judy Kingston, and included the date and time of their first meeting.[3] Twenty grandparents showed up, and the group grew from there.

Encourage Grandfathers to Come

Many grandparent groups seem to be comprised mostly of women. This is because men are traditionally less inclined to seek out self-help and support, particularly men of an older generation. Many feel they don't need to talk about their problems or believe they should be able to cope without outside help. But grandfathers do need support. Like grandmothers, they can benefit from meeting others who have similar feelings and experiences. And your group will benefit from the perspective that grandfathers offer.

When you talk to grandfathers, assure them that they are welcome and that their input is important. And then be patient. A grandmother might come alone every week for months before the grandfather comes; then one meeting might hook him. We have several men who attend meetings religiously, and their presence is always valuable. Some grandfathers even find it helps their marriage to come and learn coping skills as a couple.

Where Will You Meet?

You will need a location for your meetings. Contact churches, libraries, senior citizens' centers, schools, hospitals, and any other community buildings that have space. If you get a newspaper or radio station interested, mention that you're looking for a donated meeting room. You'll be surprised how many people in the community come through for this type of program.

Word of mouth works, too. Talk it up. Don't be afraid to tell people what you need and to ask for it! One group approached their county council of churches and found a church where they could use a kitchen and a nursery. Another grandmother attended a parenting class at her grandchild's school and received permission to use a classroom for weekly meetings. The teacher even had her class leave valentines for the grandparents who use their desks at night.

A word about chairs: Look for a room that already has chairs and/ or couches. Also try to find a variety of chairs: Some grandparents are overweight and need comfortable chairs whereas others have back problems and need sturdy support.

When Will You Meet?

Scheduling is tricky for grandparents, particularly scheduling something for themselves. Many work in the day and may not be able to find or afford a baby-sitter in the evening. Ask grandparents about times when you first contact them, and do the best you can for this first meeting. You won't please everyone, but try for a majority.

Will You Have Child Care?

From the beginning, GAP has offered child care at meetings. Many grandparents cannot afford baby-sitters and have no one to watch their grandchildren. Unless they can solve this problem, they will find it impossible to attend meetings, no matter when you schedule them. You will reach your widest population of grandparents and will be able to help the most people if you make it as easy as possible for them to attend. That means child care.

When you talk to grandparents, ask if they will need child care to attend a group meeting and, if so, how many children they will be bringing. Perhaps you or the other grandparents know someone who would be willing to baby-sit during meetings. Sometimes you can find a volunteer from a church or temple or even a college student from a local child development program who might be able to get class credit for this. One of my groups is considering rotating the responsibility among the grandparents who regularly bring grandchildren to the group meeting. (You might consider having name tags for the children so the baby-sitter can call them by name. Make sure sitters know not to release children to anyone but their grandparents.)

Will You Charge for Meetings?

I think it is critical that support groups be free of charge. Otherwise, they just become one more place where grandparents have to give. Group should be a place where they can receive. Many grandparents are on a fixed income. They don't think about their own mental health needs, they think about the needs of their grandchild. If they have an extra $60 a month, they'll buy shoes and a haircut for their grandchildren before doing anything for themselves. Charging for meetings only creates one more barrier to people receiving the help they need.

The First Meeting

Here you are. You've found a meeting place and selected the time, the kids are coloring down the hall, and you are looking at a sea of faces in front of you. You have a few more things to consider . . .

Your Panic

If you're not used to speaking in front of people, you may be nervous at this first meeting. The thoughts may tumble past, one after the other: "How do I start? What do I say? Will all the grandparents get along?" Relax. These are normal thoughts and feelings. Regardless of the group composition—age, race, income, and so on—you are all there for the same reason: You are all dealing with grandchildren in one way or another. That is the focus. This is about emotional and moral support. You are not facing strangers, you are facing future friends.

The Welcome

Introduce yourself. Welcome everyone. Restate the reason for getting together. Stress the importance of confidentiality. Share briefly about yourself: how many grandchildren you are raising, why you have them, how long you have had them, your marital status. Let others do the same. Once grandparents start talking, the group takes off.

For many grandparents, this will be their first opportunity to meet others in the same predicament and to discuss feelings and issues. There is a tremendous sense of relief the first time you walk into a room filled with people who will understand and accept you. Some, however, may not choose to talk until they feel more comfortable in the group setting. They may be perfectly happy just listening. Let them know that they are welcome even if they keep silent. And don't worry—each grandparent will wade in at his or her own pace.

Consider using name tags for this first meeting. It helps to connect names and faces in case more than a few people show up. On the other hand, don't be disappointed if you only get one or two the first night. Those two people still need help. Be patient and persistent. Some groups grow slowly, but they do grow.

Group Decisions

During this first meeting you will want to make several decisions:

▪ *Time:* Will the group keep this scheduled time? How often will it meet? I find that once a week for two to three hours works best. It depends on the number of grandparents at a given meeting—5 people can address their crises in less time than 12 people can—and on what your schedules allow. Consistency of meetings is probably more important than frequency. If the group can't meet weekly, schedule a meeting for twice a month or once a month, but make it something reliable to look forward to.

▪ *Format:* What format will you use? Will you start with all members recapping their week, or will you start with whomever is in crisis? Let the group decide what format is most comfortable, and recognize that it may change from time to time. One thing I do recommend is setting aside a few minutes for business items and announcements midway through the meeting; this way you catch people who come late and the ones who must leave early.

▪ *Time-limited or open-ended?* The majority of therapy groups are limited to a set number of weeks and don't allow new members after the first or second session. That was my plan when I started GAP. However, I soon realized that the issues grandparents encounter are much too complex and ongoing to be handled in a limited time frame. All of my groups are open-ended, with new members joining at any time. I have a policy that everyone is welcome, and I never turn anyone away. When new grandparents come into the group, they get great support and guidance from the ones who have been there longer. The grandparents are wonderful about helping each other, and that is one of the joys of the group.

▪ *Refreshments:* Will you have them? How will you handle them? If you plan to take turns, a sign-up sheet is helpful. If you prefer to pitch into a kitty with one person responsible for buying the refreshments, consider rotating the responsibility every few months.

▪ *Cleanup:* Will you have a volunteer cleanup committee to leave the room in shape? Rotate that, too.

Don't forget to have a sign-in sheet for a directory, exchange names and addresses, and keep a box of tissues handy!

Once You're Under Way

Attendance

Attendance is a changeable thing with grandparents. You will find that a core group will come to each meeting without fail. They will become your educators, helping each other out. They may even become politically active, pursuing changes that might not help their grandchildren but could save someone else's. Other grandparents will come only occasionally. Perhaps they work and can't take time off. Maybe they have medical appointments, sick grandchildren, unreliable transportation, or poor health. Encourage other members to call them and see how they're doing. Let them know they're missed.

Inevitably, a few people may drop out if this is not what they are looking for. Groups are not for everyone.

Participation

It is important that everyone at a meeting has time to share. Some grandparents may not be as verbal as others. Encourage quiet, shy grandparents to participate; as time goes by, they may become more comfortable sharing their feelings. At times, you may have to gently and politely interrupt one grandparent to give others a chance to talk.

A wonderful part of a group is that members benefit from each other's experiences, as well as from the support given and received. It's important to share positive experiences as well as negative experiences, because you learn from both.

Be Patient with Evolution

It is tempting, when you give support and advice, to push for quick changes. It is easy to become impatient with people who seem to be stuck in a situation and yet continue to suffer because of it. But change rarely comes quickly or easily, particularly where the heart is involved. Ultimately, grandparents will make the changes that they can in the time frame they can handle—and no sooner. I have heard grandparents talk for two years before they could take any action, such as getting an adult child out of the house. As a group, you can only support and encourage them. Be there when they need to cry and when they want to laugh. When they're ready to make a change, they will do it. But remember, it will be in their time frame.

There are also situations that have no answers, no clear course of action. Sometimes the only thing to do is talk, cry, and feel the understanding of people who have been there. To air your feelings, to see them as natural, and to know you're not alone and not crazy is the beginning of the healing process.

Topics

There is no standard format for subject matter in an ongoing group. Sometimes grandparents will talk about the system; sometimes they will talk about parenting issues, their own childhood, community resources, even their jobs. There is rarely an absence of topics.

(However, Appendix B offers a list of common grandparenting issues for those moments when the discussion runs dry.)

Outreach

I do a lot of outreach work. I will spend months on the phone with a grandparent in crisis; sometimes I give one grandparent the phone number of another in a similar situation. Some will eventually come out for a meeting; others will just call to hear a supportive voice.

It can be difficult to get certain grandparents to attend a group, particularly in communities that have a strong emphasis on privacy and keeping problems in the family. If you have trouble with group attendance, plan a picnic for the kids. Grandparents may not make time to come out for themselves, but they will try harder for the children.

Kicking into High Gear

Once you have a cohesive group, there are a few other things you might want to try:

Outside Experts

I have found it beneficial to occasionally invite outside experts to address my groups. Attorneys, health care specialists, and representatives from the welfare department are among those who have been kind enough to attend our meetings and share their expertise. You might also ask a local mental health professional to conduct a series of parenting classes—a lot has changed since you raised your first set of kids. But do not invite experts until your group has become a cohesive whole.

Family Activities

About once or twice a month, I plan a weekend activity that involves both grandparents and grandchildren. It is important for the children to realize that they are not alone; that many other kids are raised by grandparents; that "they're not the only ones with a Momma with gray hair," as one Grandma puts it. Group activities raise everyone's morale. We frequently have potluck picnics at a local park, reserving in advance a shelter area to guarantee some shade. Events like these give kids space to run and allow grandparents time to relax and socialize with other adults.

Donated Tickets

Many families I work with are on fixed incomes, making it difficult to do the extras they would like to do for their grandchildren. I have, on occasion, been able to obtain donated group tickets to Disneyland, Barnum and Bailey Circus, Ice Capades, Disney on Ice, local children's theaters, and various sporting events. It takes lots of phone calls and letters (often just to find out who can make the decision to donate to a group). Don't get discouraged if you ask for something and get turned down. Persistence generally does pay off.

Shared Skills

Your group is composed of grandparents who have diverse talents and abilities. You may decide to exchange these skills to help each other. For instance, in my groups I have grandparents who are willing to cut hair, repair appliances, fill out forms, and provide occasional respite care for other grandparents. Some grandparents have even volunteered to accompany each other to court. It can make you feel so much better to have someone there who cares, even when the outcome isn't positive. Exchange of these favors and services encourages mutual support.

Shared Goods

When good people come together, wonderful things happen, from clothing exchanges to acts of great generosity. Hand-me-downs were often easy pickings when you were young parents with friends who were also starting families. But when this second shift arrives late in life, you face childrearing alone—until you join a group.

One of the things my groups have organized is a clothing exchange. Grandparents bring in their grandchildren's outgrown clothing to share, and there are always families with younger grandchildren who are delighted to receive them. The same goes for toys, furniture, and other child accessories. If you do start something like this—and why not?—make sure that all donations are in good condition.

And then there is the magic . . .

When a grandfather in my group bought a new car, he and his wife donated their old one to a grandmother who didn't have one. When another grandmother could not afford to visit her dying brother, the group pooled its resources and came up with a round trip ticket to send her to see him. One grandmother was mugged immediately after cashing the check to cover her rent and food; the grandparents came to her rescue with food and donations. And a few grandparents regularly help out several families with groceries. You can't plan or schedule magic like this, it just happens. But by keeping a group together, you do set the stage for great things.

Will Your Group Need a Mental Health Professional?

One of the things you need to consider when you set up your group is if you will need a mental health professional (i.e., a social worker, psychologist, or counselor) and, if so, what his or her involvement will be.

A GAP group can work without a leader or therapist. You can become a big family, calling and supporting each other in times of stress. But there are some situations grandparents cannot cope with on their own. At some point you may have a grandparent who is in a crisis that is beyond your capacity to handle. You could, for example, have a grandparent who is suicidal and needs to be hospitalized. As a fellow grandparent, you might not know where to start. Sometimes a grandparent or grandchild needs an outside referral or needs individual therapy in addition to a self-help group. Georgia Hill is a 49-year-old grandmother who has raised her grandson since her daughter died in a car accident four years ago. A recent car accident of her own jolted her back into the grieving process, opening up all kinds of old wounds. Georgia needs more intense therapy than a group alone can provide. I referred her to someone who specializes in bereavement counseling.

I would hate for any grandparent to give improper information to another grandparent about their grandchildren, adult children, or themselves. People don't intend to hurt each other, but they can—through lack of knowledge. For example, the line between discipline and child abuse is much thinner these days than when you were raising your own children, and a lot of grandparents are capable of unwittingly giving poor advice. Washing a child's mouth out with soap, for instance, used to be a perfectly acceptable way of punishing a foul mouth; by today's standards, it is considered abusive.

It can also destroy a group if someone gives the wrong information at a meeting and it backfires. It is always better to admit you don't know something and offer to try to find out. Write down such questions and find an outside resource. Meanwhile, you might consider connecting with a mental health professional.

There are several ways a mental health professional can be involved in a GAP group:

- As a group leader
- As a regular consultant
- As an on-call consultant
- As a visiting expert

For most groups it's good to have someone on the sidelines who might not show up every week but is available to consult on complicated issues. Perhaps he or she could attend the first few meetings, while your group is becoming cohesive. At the very least, I recommend having someone do a series of classes on parenting issues. You could even arrange a group for grandchildren, who also need to know they're not alone.

How to Find a Mental Health Professional

If you are in therapy or know another grandparent in therapy, talk to the therapist. He or she may be able to recommend someone. Perhaps a local counselor or social worker is already working with three or four grandparents. Check with your local child guidance or mental health clinic for referrals. Also, any place that does outpatient therapy is a good resource.

A Word to the Mental Health Professional

Several years ago I went on vacation and left another professional to fill in for me. She couldn't wait for me to return. "All I did was answer phone calls and deal with problems," she told me. "I didn't have time to do anything else." All she saw was a group of complaining, demanding old people. She was expecting it to be easy and got a real education. If you are a professional who is considering working with a GAP group, there are two questions you need to ask yourself: Do you have a special place in your heart for this population? Do you understand how these groups differ from traditional therapy groups?

When you work with a family in outpatient therapy, you work with their mental health needs, not with the washer breaking down and the car breaking down. You may see the children in outpatient therapy for an hour a week. Grandparent groups can be much more time consuming. We are dealing with whole families and many kinds of problems, and their needs are great. GAP groups deal with more than just emotional support. From the start, my philosophy has been that if you do not deal with basic needs, you cannot begin to deal with mental health needs.

When you work with traditional therapy groups, you have rules and commitments about time, frequency, and attendance. Grandparents may show up for a group meeting once a week or once in six months; they may pop in for half an hour between doctors' appointments or before a second-shift job. They are under incredible stress, and their own care is not their first priority. They may only come when they have a crisis, or they may call regularly for advice, feedback, suggestions, and resources. I have regular contact with a lot of grandparents I never see face to face but who call when they are in need.

You do end up giving more of yourself in a GAP group than in a traditional client–therapist relationship. But if you have a feeling for grandparents, grandchildren, and their concerns, working with grandparent groups can be rewarding work.

CHAPTER 15

The Call to Action

> The seventies were a time when people became sensitive to single-parent families. Now we need awareness of a new family type—grandparents raising their grandchildren.
> —*Jessie Taylor*[1]

ere are some snapshots from the GAP political album:

Two grandmothers testify on grandparent issues before a Senate committee in Washington.[2]

Three sets of grandparents talk to Phil Donahue on national television.[3] Thousands of Americans hear what it's like to be a second-time parent.

Six grandmothers meet in chambers with a Los Angeles judge to discuss the possibility of running an information table at the county juvenile dependency courthouse. She agrees to present the idea to her colleagues.

Grandparent leaders from approximately 30 states gather at a Washington, DC, church. They are joined by representatives from the American Association of Retired Persons (AARP), the University of Pennsylvania, and the Children's Rights Council, among others. Their purpose: to explore the possibility of working as a united front. The result: the National Coalition of Grandparents (NCOG). By the end of the weekend they have drafted a mission statement and a set of goals and have elected officers.

Several hundred California grandparents and grandchildren rally on the Capitol steps in Sacramento to put faces on their issues.

And you thought you were alone . . .

The struggle to raise your grandchildren and protect their interests starts on a very personal level: in your home and in your community. This is where you juggle your schedule and your finances; where you battle social workers, judges, and sometimes your own family; where you seek out help and support. But your struggle is not taking place in a vacuum; it is part of an enormous grassroots effort fighting for grandparent and children's rights. Call it a movement. Call it a crusade. Some people call it "Granny's March on Washington." But make no mistake about it: This is not just personal, it is political.

Across the country, grandparent activists are fighting tooth and nail to protect the interests of the next generation and to make sure that future grandparents don't have to struggle so bitterly to play a part in their grandchildren's lives. Margie Davis, founder of Grandparents Offering Love and Direction (GOLD) calls it a "quiet revolution," adding, "It is one of the more important revolutions because it is changing how we care for our nation's children as well as who cares for them."[4] And it is a revolution that is getting louder.

"People think you've got to know someone or have money to get laws changed," activist grandmother Jean Churder told a reporter. "It takes complaints, and it takes people like me letting it be known. . . . A person can do a lot. Look at what one person [Candy Lightner] did with MADD [Mothers Against Drunk Driving]."[5] Jean is a grandmother of 13 and founder of Grandparents and Grandchildren, a political action group in Riverside, California. An assembly speaker accidentally referred to her as "Mrs. Rock" after she described grandparents as the Rock of Gibraltar in their grandchildren's lives. That nickname would also be appropriate for the grandparent activists I work with. They are committed to seeing change. They work at all levels of activism, from facilitating support groups to traveling to Washington, DC, for Senate hearings. They meet with supervisors, judges, and social service agencies; serve on the executive committees of state and national coalitions; and have been a resource to grandparents all across the United States. Each one is like my right arm; I know I can rely on them.

HISTORY OF GRANDPARENTS' RIGHTS MOVEMENT

The idea of grandparents' rights is not a new concept. As far back as 1894 a Louisiana grandmother petitioned the courts for the right to visit her grandchildren.[6] What is new is how widespread the fight has become. The first generation of grandparent activists started in the mid-1960s. They were mostly third parties in custody battles and mostly unrecognized by the courts, and they generated attention and debate on one central issue: grandparent visitation.[7] These grandparents fought social workers, lawyers, and local lawmakers across the country, spurring the first grandparent statutes in a number of states. By the middle of the '80s all 50 states (but not the District of Columbia) had a grandparent visitation statute on their books.

The first wave of grandparent activism also caught the attention of Congress. Although Congress has no legislative authority over family law, it can pass "sense of Congress" resolutions, a kind of formal recommendation to the states. In 1985 former Congressman Mario Biaggi (D–NY) introduced a resolution (H. Con. Res. 67) recommending that all states adopt uniform grandparent visitation laws—in the case of death, divorce, or dissolution of marriage of the parents. The resolution passed unanimously, although state action is slow in coming.[8]

Then, in the late '80s a new generation of grandparents hit the streets. They don't just want to *see* their grandchildren, they are raising them. And they are lighting political fires to protect their interests. They have formed support groups—with names like Grandparents United for Children's Rights, Grandparents Raising Grandchildren, Grandparents Reaching Out, and my own Grandparents As Parents (GAP)—and are pursuing not only visitation issues but issues of custody, government aid, and even the very definition of *family* in today's society. "Network!" is their rallying cry. They network in their own communities with sympathetic judges, lawyers, lawmakers, and social services personnel; with other grandparent groups through state and national coalitions; and with congresspeople and senators by participating in state and federal hearings.

This generation of grandparents is educating themselves about the system so they can work through the system. "Until 15 years ago, people were in awe of legislation," says Ethel Dunn, executive director of Grandparents United for Children's Rights. "Now they see that it's just a law, and we can change it." They are also educating the system about themselves and their issues. "The granny in the sensible shoes and blue hair—you don't see her anymore," says Dunn.[9]

Much of this book has been about loss and stark realities. There is no question that you have been dealt a mean hand in this game, and the stakes are high against you. But this book is also about hope and the difference one person can make. One person, a grandparent, makes an enormous difference in the life of a neglected child. One person who starts a group helps each person who joins it. And one person joining forces with another person, and another, and another can changes laws and move mountains. "The only way to make any changes in children's rights is for us to find each other and help each other," says Barbara Kirkland, founder of Grandparents Raising Grandchildren.[10]

You do have power. I know it is hard to believe, especially when a nameless, faceless welfare worker cuts your benefits or a harsh judge gives unsupervised visitation to your abusive son-in-law. But as a group you have clout. "Supervisors are afraid of people like you," says attorney Michael Salazar. "You're the ones who vote. You've got the country on the run, under tremendous political pressure."[11] Former Congressman Thomas Downey (D–NY) would agree. "It's a well known fact that seniors are the most active lobby in the country," he said in a 1991 congressional hearing. "And when it comes to grandparents, there is no one group more united in their purpose."[12]

Strength in numbers. Unity. That is your power. It is surprising how few letters or phone calls it takes to make legislators look at something. They get no feedback on most of what they work on, so it doesn't take much mail to make something an issue. And people in government do listen. Already we are making headway, and every victory is a milestone! Here are some of our achievements:

▪ *States are beginning to understand that grandparents do have a role to play in the family.* Visitation statutes are being tested, state by state and even at the U.S. Supreme Court level. Some states even have "intact family" bills, which allow grandparents to petition for visitation even though the parents are still married.[13] Arizona allows grandparents to petition even if the parents were never married.[14] Nevada passed a law in 1991 giving grandparents and other relatives preference for child placement even when they live outside the state.[15] Texas grandparents who have guardianship of their grand-children may include them on their group health insurance.[16] Maine passed a bill in 1994 that gives grandparents the right to petition for standing in child protection proceedings.[17]

• *Communications are improving between grandparents, social workers, and the courts.* GOLD has worked with the San Diego County Department of Social Services to establish an information table at the San Diego courthouse. It is staffed by trained grandparent volunteers and offers court-approved information from GOLD and other groups. According to Margie Davis, founder of GOLD, the judges, attorneys, and social workers all love it.[18]

• *We have the ear of legislators.* Ethel Dunn and I get calls from various local and state senators asking for feedback on legislation. I have even had three-way conference calls with local senate aides and the American Bar Association in Washington, DC, to change the language of a proposed bill.

• *We have the attention of congresspeople and senators.* From 1990 to 1992 grandparents testified before three congressional hearings on the issues of grandparents and children, including the first Senate hearing on the subject.[19]

• *The National Coalition of Grandparents (NCOG) was formed.* I don't think there is a better signal to grandparents that your voice will be heard, and with groups constantly cropping up in different states, our ranks keep growing.

• *Local coalitions are on the rise.* Support groups in several areas have begun to network and organize themselves to create a stronger voice on local issues. California has a statewide coalition of grandparent and relative caregivers; Washington, Oregon, and Idaho have created a tristate coalition; and similar efforts are taking place in other regions of the country.[20]

• *We have a national resource center.* In 1993 the American Association of Retired Persons created the AARP Grandparent Information Center in Washington, DC. The center is a clearinghouse for national and local resources. It includes a database of hundreds of grandparent support groups across the country and received 2,100 calls for information in its first four months of operation alone.[21]

These are all signs of progress. Still, NCOG copresident Ethel Dunn cautions patience. "Individually, when you talk to grandparents, they'll be very frustrated. They're not winning their case now, and they see the clock ticking; they recognize that their grandchildren are losing time with them, and they are losing time with their grandkids. But in the overall sense, grandparents are making headway. We're gaining respectability."[22] It is that very frustration itself that drives people into the grandparent movement. Political action gives them a place to channel their anger and their energy. "You feel as though you're doing something," she explains. "You're not sitting and wallowing in your pain."

"This has become a passion with me," says GAP member Barbara Wasson. "When I got involved I thought that the state protected children. I found out the state does not protect them. I want to be a part of helping these children have a voice, with education, changing laws, whatever it takes."[23]

Rosalie Cauley no longer has her grandson with her; he was returned to his mother by a dependency judge. Still, Rosalie is a staunch advocate for grandparents' and children's rights. "When Jeremy was first taken, we were absolutely devastated," she explains. "We didn't know what to do with our time or our energy, where to put all this anger. We wanted to work towards improving the system and protecting children. We have told Jeremy that we may not be able to help him, but maybe some other little kid won't have to go through what he's gone through."[24]

LIGHTING THE POLITICAL TORCH

Don't let the word *political* scare you. There are many ways to make a difference without actually rallying on the Capitol steps—although some of our grandparents found that to be an exciting experience. You can work behind the scenes with legislators by sponsoring a bill, shaping a bill, or just supporting it with calls and letters. You can work with judges, attorneys, and social workers, offering them resources and educating them about your concerns. You can work with the media and the community, creating public awareness and public education about children's rights and grandparents' rights. But if you do want to impact policy, you need to be armed with knowledge about the issues, the process of government, and the players. You need to make yourself heard.

Know the Issues

To be taken seriously, you have to know your subject: the history of the issue, the stories, the statistics, anything that will make your concerns real to the people who can help you. If you can do this and be specific, detailed, and well organized with your information, you will have a valuable perspective to offer those you are working with.

You must also know the bills. Is there something already under consideration? It may need your support—perhaps a letter to your legislator or your testimony at a hearing. Is this a new area that needs to be introduced to your legislators? You may want to provide model bills from other states or join forces with a politically savvy attorney who can work with legislative offices to draft a new bill. Many attorneys feel strongly about issues like children's rights and kinship care; perhaps you can work with one who is willing to volunteer the time.

Trust what you know. Many grandparents assume that they are only "bumbling little grannies" and that other people know more than they do. As they move forward, they discover they have a wealth of information and insight to offer.

Know the Process

Before you can fight the system, or even work within it, you must know how it works—not just the courts and the agencies but the workings of your local, state, and federal governments as well. You know what the problems are, but who causes them? Where do they start? Who can change them? Is the problem one of process or one of law? It makes a difference. "Trial judges and jurors must interpret the laws as written by legislators," a California court judge told us. In other words, don't picket the court, picket the capitol. Is it a federal issue or a local one? Most issues that are important to grandparents originate at the state and local levels. It's not worth sending thousands of letters to a federal representative when it is a local law in question.

Know the Players

Political advocacy is a big field with many issues and just as many players. Some people can help you, others cannot. You need to know the difference. Who is on your side—and can you work together? Who is against you—and can you sway them? Who is undecided? To answer these questions you need to know the following groups:

▪ *Your representatives:* Do you know who your council member is? Your delegate in Congress? Your state senator or assembly member? These are the people most likely to listen to you. You are one of the people they were elected to serve, and you are one of those who will keep them in office. Your concerns should be their concerns. But before you contact them, here are some things you might want to know about them: their concerns and interests, their voting record on family issues, the stands they are taking now, and the committees they serve on. The more you know in advance about your representatives, the better you can focus your appeal. After all, you will approach a sympathetic listener differently than someone who is antagonistic or on the fence.

▪ *Your allies:* Few issues exist in a vacuum. For every issue that you promote or oppose, there is probably another group working with the same agenda. For instance, Grandparents United for Children's Rights joined forces with the National Foster Parents Association to support a national kinship mandate;[25] both groups would like to see a uniform law requiring all child welfare agencies to look to family members before placing a child in unrelated foster care. Whatever your goal, network with other groups in your area. Find out who shares your position and whether you can work together. At least make sure you don't double someone else's efforts. Remember, numbers count. A coalition has more clout than one grandparent or even one group alone.

There are many groups that keep an eye on family and child legislation; the Foster Parent Association, Children Now, Child Welfare League, and the National Association of Social Workers are just a few. Many of these groups have state chapters. Your group could join forces with one of them, and their newsletters are a good way to follow current developments.

▪ *Your opposition:* It's great to sit and agree with your friends, but at some point you have to turn and face your enemies. Every issue you support may have someone who opposes it; the more you know about them, the better chance you have of answering their arguments, perhaps even of swaying them to your side. Be willing to negotiate.

Make Yourself Heard!

None of your passion or knowledge will help your cause if no one hears about it. Don't just tell your friends and neighbors, tell your government officials. If they are to represent you, they must know how issues and actions affect you. They have the clout to make the changes.

Letter Writing

Letters do count. Legislators don't get tired of hearing from their constituents. Legislators read their mail, and what they read can affect their position on a bill or issue. Remember, most bills don't get any letters at all, so a little mail goes a long way.

One California grandmother wrote a letter that was so eloquent it was copied into every senator's folder as part of the legislative analysis of the bill it was supporting. "That's history here in the Senate," says legislative assistant Leza Davis. "Five years from now, if someone wants to get the bill folder from the archives, they will see Rosalie's letter."[26] Incidentally, the bill passed. So don't think your letter is unimportant. This is a case of the squeaky wheel getting the grease—if it is handled properly.

Who Should Get Your Letter?

Knowing where to send a letter sounds simple, but you'd be surprised at how many people write letters to officials who can't help them. A well-targeted letter does more good than randomly papering your capitol with mail. Here are some suggestions to help you target your letters:

▪ *Write to your own representatives.* You have more influence with senators from your state and representatives from your district than with anyone else. Give them your support if they agree with you. If they don't, explain why a different position makes sense right now. Show your familiarity with the issue, and cite your firsthand experience.

▪ *Write to the relevant committee members.* If you have facts you think should influence their thinking, send them to the chairperson

How to Write Effective Political Letters*

1. Begin with the appropriate heading and address. Elected officials are addressed as "The Honorable," followed by their name. In the letter use the proper title: "Dear Senator Jones," "Dear Assembly Member Thomas," "Dear Congressman Smith," "Dear Governor Jackson."

2. Be specific. State the actual bill number, if you can, or at least provide the bill's title.

3. State your opinion in the first sentence.

4. Identify yourself and explain why you are concerned about this issue. Give factual information to support your view. If you are writing on behalf of a group, include the group's name and the size of its membership—there is strength in numbers.

5. State how this bill will address the problem and how it will affect your district.

6. Close by urging your representative to take appropriate, specific action.

7. Sign your name legibly and include your address on the letter itself; sometimes envelopes get lost or pitched.

8. Include any pertinent materials, for example, editorials from local papers.

Remember to . . .

- Write about one subject only.
- Be brief and to the point; one page should do it.
- Write legibly, or type if you can. But don't put off writing just because you don't type; every letter counts.
- Use your own words instead of a form letter. Use your own stationary, unless you are writing on behalf of a group or organization (then use the organization letterhead).
- Keep letters individual. If you write several legislators, don't send identical letters. And don't send photocopied letters, form letters, or printed post cards.
- Be courteous and reasonable.

A Few Don'ts

- Don't be self-righteous. Your legislators know you are a citizen and a taxpayer; you don't have to flaunt it.

(continued)

(continued from previous page)

- Don't apologize for taking your legislator's time. Just be concise and specific.
- Don't make comments like "I hope this gets by your secretary." This only irritates and alienates office staff.
- Don't be rude or threatening.
- Don't be vague.

---

*Adapted from "A Walk through Policyland" by Grandparents United for Children's Rights.

or the members of a committee that will hear a bill. If you do this, send a copy to your own legislator with a short personal note.

- *Don't complain to legislators from other districts.* Just because you disagree politically with your own legislators does not mean that it is a good idea to write to a member of another district. Write to your legislator directly.
- *Write to the fence-sitters.* Before a bill goes to vote, find out who is on your side and who is not. You have a better chance of swaying the ones who are undecided than in reversing the position of someone who is dead-set against you.
- *Write to the governor.* Even if a state bill passes both houses, the governor will still have to sign it. But don't wait for a bill to reach the governor's desk before starting your letter-writing campaign.

When to Write

Timing is critical when you are writing political action letters. Whether you are writing to propose, support, or oppose a bill, you want to make sure your letter arrives at the right stage of the process to be effective. Here are some general guidelines on timing:

- To propose a bill or submit ideas for legislation, write during your state's legislative recess. This gives the staff time to research your issue.
- To affect the writing and language of a bill, write when it is being considered in committee.
- To advocate for or against a bill, write at the beginning of committee hearings if your representative is on the committee; if not, write just before the bill comes to the floor.

▪ If the bill has passed both houses, write to your governor. Make sure your letter goes out early enough to be considered; this is your last chance for input.

When time is of the essence, you can send a telegram or Mailgram or even make a phone call or send a fax to your official's office. If enough calls come in, he or she will get the message. Your public officials also need positive feedback. Write to let them know when they've done a good job for you, not just to complain or to oppose their actions.

Working with Legislators

If you want to influence the writing of new laws, you will want to establish a relationship with your public officials. Once you do that, you can educate them about your concerns and position yourself as a reliable sounding board for grandparent issues. Lawmakers can't possibly know every implication of the laws they write; they must rely on outside experts. You can get to know your legislators by inviting them to one of your meetings or by scheduling private appointments with them. Don't be discouraged if you start out meeting with their aides. Aides and consultants are good people to know. They are advisers and often gather information for their senator, representative, or council member.

The Visit

When you visit a legislator in his or her office, try to be as organized and professional as possible. Remember that legislators must make time in a busy schedule to see you, and let them know that you know their time is valuable by arriving early and keeping your meeting brief. Be honest and courteous; remember, you are trying to create a relationship with this person, not just win one vote. Some other techniques for an effective visit include the following:

▪ *Be prepared and be concise.* Have your information ready ahead of time and get to the point quickly; keep your presentation simple and specific.
▪ *Bring a written position paper.* Writing it will focus your thoughts, and it gives you something to leave with your legislator.

- *Keep your group small.* Too many people with too many voices can overwhelm a person and dilute your message.
- *Offer solutions.* "[Lawmakers] don't have time to solve your problems for you," says GOLD founder Margie Davis.[27] "Never take a problem without a solution."
- *Avoid arguments.* You want your legislator to see the issues from your perspective, you don't want to create an adversary. Be composed, not confrontational.
- *Avoid war stories.* You want your legislator to see this issue as one that affects more than one grandparent. You can do this by showing the broad picture, not your personal story. "You watch sometime," says one grandparent activist. "If you're with an official and a grandmother starts talking about 'My granddaughter . . . ,' you can see the curtain close, and they're not listening."[28] If you want to be heard, stay impersonal.
- *Always end your visit with a question.* For example: "Will you support this issue?" "What can you do to help us?" Grandparent issues need legislative support; don't be afraid to come out and ask for it.
- *Don't forget to thank your legislator for his or her time.*
- *Remeber to follow up your visit with a letter.* Remind your public official of any commitment he or she made and express your gratitude yet again for his or her time and support.

Step by Step

Remember, each piece of legislation is a step, not a cure. This is a slow process, and not every effort will succeed. But even small changes make a big difference. You don't always need to write a new law; you can help change (or enforce) existing laws. For instance, a Virginia grandmother and foster parent wanted to help change foster care laws in her state. She took one issue—the amount of time children remain in the foster care system—and worked with her state legislature. She was persistent, organized, and diplomatic. Today, a child can be in the Virginia foster care system no more than two years, instead of five, before a permanent plan is established.[29]

Expect changes in your original amendments. Your public officials are trying to balance the concerns of many people, departments, and interest groups at the same time. Be willing to work with your opponents and stay open to discussion. You might end up with a better product. And don't forget: Each grandparent situation is different. Many issues will continue to be decided court by court and case by case. Legislators write laws, but judges still interpret them.

Public Awareness and Political Education

Political action goes beyond writing and rewriting legislation. Laws must be passed, they must be interpreted, and they must be carried out. While it is important to work with legislators, for real change to come about you must also educate the people who vote on, interpret, and execute new legislation. The trick is to know your audience and how to approach them.

Judges and Attorneys

Like legislators, judges and attorneys are not able to keep track of all issues that affect their work. They need outside sources of information—but these need to be impersonal sources. It doesn't do to approach these professionals with your own story and needs; they can't address individual cases, and they will, unfortunately, stop listening to you. You can set up an office visit with a judge, but, as with a lawmaker, be sure to come in representing the larger issues and don't bring a problem without a proposed solution. The basic question you are posing is "How can we work together?"

You can also try tapping into continuing education. Judges and attorneys must earn a certain number of educational credits a year to keep up with new trends. Grandparent issues definitely present a new trend in law. A well-organized grandparent group could offer to create a panel of grandparents and legal experts for one of these educational programs. This may take some salesmanship and advance planning, but it offers you a chance to educate decision makers in a nonthreatening environment. Remember, however, that your goal is to educate, not complain.

Social Services and Social Workers

The more thoroughly social workers can understand the plight of grandparents in general—outside their individual caseload—the better chance they have of being sensitized to grandparent issues. Working with local legislators, attorneys, and activists in children's rights and foster parent organizations will bring you into networking contact with social service administrators; you can also contact them directly. Again, position yourself as a positive resource.

The Media

The media is on a constant hunt for human interest stories. As grandparents raising grandchildren, your stories are lightning rods for many social ills. This is one place where individual details and strong emotions are appropriate. Remember, the media shapes public opinion, and public opinion shapes government.

DOWN THE ROAD: REDEFINING THE FAMILY

Family renification and parental rights are the key stumbling blocks you encounter as a grandparent with a grandchild in crisis. The courts are pledged to support family reunification, and parental rights are closely guarded. These are important ideals. The problems don't lie with the importance our society attaches to family and parents, the problems lie with the definition of *family* and *parent*.

For centuries the family was a wide net that included grandparents, uncles, aunts, cousins, even great-grandparents. Today, however, law and society define family in the narrowest of terms: mother, father, and child. When the law breaks the relationship between a parent and child, all of the child's other blood ties cease to exist. This kind of thinking is absurd. To quote psychiatrist Arthur Kornhaber, M.D., "Nature doesn't limit the family to two generations; why should the law?"[30]

The concept of parent is even more complicated. Traditionally, parents gave birth to a child and then raised him. Today, increasing numbers of children are raised by stepparents, foster parents, adoptive parents, grandparents, and other relatives—people who have no direct biological connection to the child but have cared for and bonded with him on a day-to-day basis. Still, we repeatedly see the courts take a child away from one parent, place him with relatives, and then go looking for the "real" father or mother—whether that person knows the child or not. Some grandparents angrily refer to these absent parents as "sperm donors" and "egg carriers," but the law remains on their side.

We need to redefine the word *parent,* and we need to consider more than biology in our definition. Until we do, we can expect more and more painful battles between parents and grandparents, between biological and foster parents, and between adoptive parents and birth mothers. The advent of artificial insemination, *in vitro* fertilization, surrogate motherhood, and test-tube babies raises whole new questions about parenthood. As one scientist told GOLD founder Margie Davis, "If those in the social service end of the world do not redefine the word *parent,* we in the scientific community will do it for you."[31] The grandparent movement, by its very existence, is helping to broaden the definitions of parent and family. With every lawsuit, with every hearing, with every magazine article, grandparents and other child advocates are informing the public about parenthood and family issues. Only through education, discussion, and public acceptance will true change occur.

Remember, anyone can make a baby. It takes a parent to raise a child.

CHAPTER 16

Conclusion

> You know they say blood is thicker than water?
> Well, for us, love is thicker than blood.
> —*Jonathan Williams, 37, raised by*
> *step-grandmother and grandfather*[1]

In an issue of "The Intergenerational Hookup," the newsletter of Grandparents United for Children's Rights, executive director Ethel Dunn wrote a moving article about Las Madres de la Plaza de Mayo (the mothers of the Plaza de Mayo). These were the middle- and upper-class mothers and grandmothers of Argentina who gathered each Thursday in the square outside Argentina's White House to protest the disappearance of thousands of children and grandchildren during the military government's campaign against "subversives" in the mid-1970s and early 1980s. As many as 4,000 of these children were believed to have been kidnapped and turned over to military families for adoption. These grieving mothers and grandmothers translated their fear into anger and their anger into advocacy; they walked in a large silent circle, week after week, carrying pictures of missing children. It is a story of courage, love, and determination.

In our own country there is no military government spiriting away children. But since the 1980s the threat of drugs and alcohol, violent crime, child abuse, AIDS, and a bureaucratic court system have endangered far more than 4,000 children. Here, too, there are thousands of grandparents who are turning grief and fear into advocacy. "Sometimes we, too, march, picket, carry signs, and demand," writes Dunn. "We never stop trying to educate. We sometimes become angry, often frustrated. Once in a while we smell the passionate fragrance of success and allow ourselves a short period of time to rejoice. Always, however, we persevere."[2]

Persevere. It means to continue in spite of difficulty and opposition. It doesn't matter if you are on a picket line or in a grocery line; every grandparent trying to raise a grandchild perseveres. Each morning your grandchildren wake up safe and each night they go to bed well loved and well cared for, you have succeeded. Each grandparent who has lost a grandchild perseveres, and each day that grandparent survives the sorrow, he or she has succeeded.

Grandparents in Los Angeles, California, and Paducah, Kentucky, have as much to tell about courage, love, and determination as Las Madres de la Plaza de Mayo. If you ever wonder where the rewards come from, consider the following letter, which was written by my nephew Kevin, now in college.[3] It is addressed to my mother, the grandmother who raised him:

Nona,

On July 31st, 1983, you unexpectedly became a mother again. You took an 8-year-old boy into your home and treated him like he was your son, as if it was normal.

Your life was turned upside down. You lost the most precious thing in the world to you—your daughter. In the middle of your pain and suffering you found the time to take care of a scared, confused, and uncertain little boy who had just lost his mother.

As the little boy got older, he learned how to push your buttons. He had a knack for making your day miserable. Making life hard for you was his way of saying he didn't want another mom. He did everything he could to push you away, but you wouldn't leave him alone. The more problems he caused, the more you were there for him—getting him out of trouble and pushing him to do something with his life. You never thought twice about helping him when he needed it. When he was sick, you nursed him back to health. When he wanted a ride to a friend's house, you took him there. You always tried your hardest to make him happy.

Now he has grown up and understands the sacrifices you made for him.

Nona, this little boy is a very grateful young man now, and I want you to know how much I appreciate all you've done for me.

I want you to know that I'm proud to be your grandson. But most of all, I want you to know I love you.

Kevin

The great American poet Carl Sandburg once said, "A baby is God's opinion that the world should go on." When you take in a grandchild, you do more than help one family; you preserve our future.

Appendices

Resources for Grandparents and Relative Caregivers

FOR FINDING GROUPS IN YOUR AREA

AARP Grandparent Information Center
AARP Headquarters
601 E St., N.W.
Washington, DC 20049
(202) 434-2296 Weekdays, 9:00 A.M. to 5:00 P.M. EST

You can write to them or call. If you call, you will hear a recorded message asking for your name and phone number. Center staff will return your call, keeping your expense to a minimum.

Grandparents As Parents (GAP)
P.O. Box 964
Lakewood, CA 90714
(310) 924-3996
(310) 839-2548
Fax: (714) 828-1375

Grandparents United for Children's Rights
137 Larkin St.
Madison, WI 53705
(608) 238-8751

SOURCES OF ADDITIONAL SUPPORT

Al-Anon (also Alateen and Alatot)
Al-Anon Family Group Headquarters
P.O Box 862
Midtown Station, NY 10018-0862
(212) 302-7240

You can also look up Al-Anon in your telephone book for information on local groups.

Compassionate Friends
P.O. Box 3696
Oakbrook, IL 60522-3696
(708) 990-0010

This is a group for bereaved parents who have lost children of any age, for any reason.

PARENTING RESOURCES

American Council for Drug Education
204 Monroe St., Suite 110
Rockville, MD 20850
(800) 488-DRUG

Boy Scouts of America
1325 W. Walnut Hill Lane
Irving, TX 75015-2079
(214) 580-2000

This organization can work with learning disabled children. It also runs a major antidrug program, which includes the publication of a booklet for children.

Children and Adults with Attention Deficit Disorder (CHADD)
499 N.W. 70th Ave., Suite 109
Plantation, FL 33317
(800) 233-4050
Fax: (305) 587-4599

Educational Resources Information Center (ERIC) System
1600 Research Blvd.
Rockville, MD 20850-3172
(800) 538-3742

ERIC is a promotional and outreach arm of the U.S. Department of Education's Office of Educational Research and Improvement. It offers free materials on topics like "How Can I Be Involved in My Child's Education?" It publishes a free education journal, *The ERIC Review*, three times a year. Call for a subscription or to order free brochures.

Learning Disabilities Association (LDA)
4156 Library Rd.
Pittsburgh, PA 15234
(412) 341-1525

This association is for children and adults with learning disabilities.

Mothers Against Drunk Driving (MADD)
511 E. John Carpenter Freeway, Suite 700
Irving, TX 75062
(214) 744-6233

In addition to legislative action, MADD offers programs to help young children develop positive self-esteem and refusal skills.

National Association for Perinatal Addiction Research and Education (NAPARE)
200 N. Michigan Ave., Suite 300
Chicago, IL 60601
(800) 638-2229

In addition to its national help line, NAPARE offers free information on caring for drug-exposed children. Ask for their *Foster Parent* and *Adoptive Parent* packets.

National Clearinghouse for Alcohol and Drug Information
11426-28 Rockville Pike
Rockville, MD 20852
(800) 729-6686

This is a federal clearinghouse that provides pamphlets, booklets, posters, fact sheets, and directories on alcohol and drugs.

National Information Center for Children and Youth with Disabilities (NICHCY)
P.O. Box 1492
Washington, DC 20013
(800) 695-0285

NICHCY is a clearinghouse for free information on disabilities and disability-related issues involving children and youth. NICHCY publications include explanations of special education laws and school services for children with disabilities, state resource sheets, and information on individual disabilities. Some materials are printed in Spanish. Call or write NICHCY for a free copy of their publications list.

National Institute on Drug Abuse (NIDA)
5600 Fishers Lane
Rockville, MD 20857
(800) 729-6686

NIDA provides drug information and a counseling hotline.

National PTA Drug and Alcohol Abuse Prevention Project
330 N. Wabash Ave., Suite 2100
Chicago, IL 60611-3690
(312) 670-6782

Open Arms Family Support Network
P.O. Box 50982
Pasadena, CA 91115-0982
(818) 383-6800

Publishes the *Open Arms Baby Book: Special Care Techniques for Infants Prenatally Exposed to Drugs or Alcohol.* Available by mail for a $2.00 donation.

CHILD-FOCUSED BOOKS

Ages Four to Eight

Do I Have a Daddy? (Jeanne Warren Lindsay). Buena Park, CA: Morning Glory, 1991. Age level: five to eight years old. This story provides a model for how to respond to children's questions about a parent they have never seen.

Nonna (Jennifer Bartoli). New York, NY: Harvey House, 1975. Age level: four to seven years old. A boy tells the story of the death of his grandmother, portraying how young children respond to the death of a loved one.

The Saddest Time (Norma Simon). Morton Grove, IL: Whitman, Albert & Co., 1986. Age level: four to eight years old. Death is the subject of these three gentle stories.

When Grandpa Died (Margaret Stevens). Chicago, IL: Children's Press, 1979. Age level: four to eight years old. A little girl learns to accept the death of her grandfather.

Ages Eight to 13

Aarvy Aardvark Finds Hope (Donna O'Toole). Burnsville, NC: Celo Press, 1988. Age level: all ages. An aardvark's delayed grief over the loss of family begins to heal through the support of a caring friend.

Blew and the Death of the Mag (Wendy Lichtman). Albion, CA: Freestone, 1975. Age level: 10 and up. After her mother dies, a young girl explores her feelings of love, fear, anger, and, finally, understanding.

How It Feels When a Parent Dies (Jill Krementz). New York, NY: Alfred A. Knopf, 1981. Eighteen children, ages seven through 16, tell how it feels to lose a parent through death.

Older Children

Unlocking Potential: College and Other Choices for Learning Disabled People— A Step-By-Step Guide (Barbara Scheiber and Jeane Talpers). Chevy Chase, MD: Adler & Adler, 1987. Available only through Woodbine House, 6510 Bells Mill, Bethesda, MD 20817. (800) 843-7323. $12.95 plus $4.00 shipping/handling.

LEGAL ORGANIZATIONS AND ASSOCIATIONS

American Bar Association
750 N. Lake Shore
Chicago, IL 60611
(312) 988-5000

Legal Services for Prisoners with Children
474 Valencia St., Suite 230
San Francisco, CA 94103
(415) 255-7036

This organization publishes several state manuals for grandparent/relative caregivers and their advocates.

National Association of Protection and Advocacy Systems
900 Second St., N.E., Suite 211
Washington, DC 20002
(202) 408-9514

Protection and advocacy agencies pursue legal, administrative, and other solutions to protect the rights of people who are developmentaly disabled or mentally ill.

LEGAL BOOKS AND PUBLICATIONS

Family Law Dictionary (Robin D. Leonard and Stephen Elias). Berkeley, CA: Nolo Press, 1990.

The Guardianship Book: How to Become a Child's Guardian in California (David Brown). Berkeley, CA: Nolo Press, 1989.

POLITICAL ACTION RESOURCES

American Association of Retired Persons (AARP)
AARP Headquarters
601 E St., N.W.
Washington, DC 20049
(202) 434-2296 Weekdays, 9:00 A.M. to 5:00 P.M. EST

National Coalition of Grandparents (NCOG)
137 Larkin St.
Madison, WI 53705
(608) 238-8751

Western Union
(800) 325-6000

Western Union has a reduced rate for messages to public officials. Personal Opinion Messages (POMs) carry a flat rate for 20 words and will reach your legislator in one day. The voice response system will prompt you through the various choices.

Conversation Topics
for Grandparent
Support Groups

THE STORIES

- How many grandchildren you have and how you came to have them.

LIFE CHANGES

- The decrease in your social life now that you're a parent again
- How your life is different from that of your friends
- How your grandchildren have changed your work life
- Your feelings about work
- The financial strain of raising a second family
- The dreams and plans that have been put on hold
- The toll on your health

INTENSE FEELINGS

- Grief over the loss of your child
- Anger at your child, the situation, the system, everything
- Guilt
- Depression
- Feeling you don't want to raise your grandchildren, but not wanting them split up or placed with strangers
- Feeling you don't belong anywhere, neither with young parents nor with adults your age

- Fears
- Hopes for your grandchildren
- The small rewards

PARENTING ISSUES

- Changes in childrearing techniques since you brought up your own kids
- The effects of the parent's visits on the child's behavior and emotions
- Dealing with school problems children might have
- Setting limits with grandchildren and adult children; what behaviors you will or will not tolerate
- Setting age-appropriate consequences
- How to raise your grandchild's self-esteem
- How to help children who were born drug exposed
- Learning to accept that some grandchildren might need more help than you can provide

YOUR ADULT CHILDREN

- Learning to accept the fact that your son or daughter is choosing to be an irresponsible parent
- When to decide that you have done enough for your adult child and that it's time to let go
- Protecting yourself and your grandchildren from your adult child

THE REST OF YOUR FAMILY

- The reaction of other children and family members to your becoming a parent again
- Handling sibling rivalry
- The effects of second parenthood on your marriage

THE BUREAUCRACY

- How to negotiate the bureaucracy of government agencies and "the system"

- The frustration with a system that was set up to protect your grand-children but often doesn't
- What groups can do to help change the system

A Guide to the Grandparents Mentioned in This Book

Liz Andersson, in her 70s, raising five grandsons, ages 18 months to 12 years, in Seattle, Washington

Rose and Gerald Avery, in their 50s, raising two grandsons in Boston, Massachusetts

Janet Baker, in her 50s, raising three granddaughters in Los Angeles, California

Jewell Baxter, in her 60s, raising two grandsons, ages three and four, in Anaheim, California

Alice Brody, in her 60s, raising three grandchildren in Wilmington, Delaware

Marjorie Brown, in her 40s, raising three-year-old Jessica and two-year-old Billy in Chicago, Illinois

Charlotte Buckley, in her 40s, raising four-year-old Joey in Los Angeles, California

Maggie Butler, in her 50s, raising two granddaughters in Columbus, Ohio

Henrietta Casper, in her 70s, raising 15-year-old Adam in Long Beach, California

Ruth Castle, in her 60s, raising two grandsons in Los Angeles, California

Rosalie Cauley, in her 50s, lives in Lakewood, California, and is no longer raising 14-year-old Jeremy

Sandra Cobb, in her 60s, raising seven grandchildren in Washington, D.C.

Katherine Connor, in her 60s, raising five grandchildren in Long Beach, California

Leah Croft, in her 60s, raising nine-year-old twins and three-year-old Josh in Woodland Hills, California

Lucy Davis, in her 50s, raising seven-year-old Lindsey in Studio City, California

Wanda Davis, in her 50s, raising eight-year-old Monica in Tuscon, Arizona

Andre and Ginette de Toledo, in their 60s, raised 19-year-old Kevin in Culver City, California

Barbara Douglas, in her 80s, raising eight-year-old Max in Warwick, Rhode Island

Beth and Alan Grafton, in their 60s, raising three grandchildren in Boston, Massachusetts

Joyce Griffin, in her 60s, raising five grandchildren in Houston, Texas

Nancy Harper, in her 50s, raising eight-year-old Marissa in Los Angeles, California

Georgia Hill, in her 40s, raising seven-year-old Stephen in Long Beach, California

Marlena Hunt, in her 40s, raising two-year-old Tiffany in Anaheim, California

Ivy Johnson, in her 50s, raising five grandchildren in Baltimore, Maryland

Dorcas King, in her 70s, raising two grandchildren in Los Angeles, California

Victor Lane, in his 60s, raising three grandchildren in Long Beach, California

Pam and Robert Marshall, in their 60s, raising five-year-old Megan in Long Beach, California

Frances Morgan, in her 70s, raising two grandchildren in Tarzana, California

Ethel Murray, in her 70s, raising nine-year-old Scott in Springfield, Illinois

Carolyn Parker, in her 50s, raising six-year-old Eric in Los Angeles, California

Emily and Carter Petersen, in their 60s, raising four-year-old Amanda and three-year-old Jared in Buffalo, New York

Claire and Evan Powers, in their 60s, in Santa Monica, California, no longer raising 12-year-old Sarah, but see her one weekend a month

Sue Ellen Rice, in her 50s, raising four-year-old Martin and two-year-old Alice in San Diego, California

Jay and Brenda Saunders, in their 70s, raising six-year-old Anthony in Hartford, Connecticut

Jack and Betty Segal, in their 60s, raising eight-year-old Beth in Portland, Oregon

Frank and Gloria Simon, in their 60s, raising eight-year-old Stephanie and six-year-old Jill in Los Angeles, California

Donna and Hal Smith, in their 50s, raising ten-year-old David and six-year-old John in Sacramento, California

Esther Smith, in her 80s, in Scottsdale, Arizona, no longer has her grandsons living with her

Diane Snyder, in her 50s, raising seven-year-old Andrea in Azuza, California

Marta Sobol, in her 50s, raising eight-year-old Christopher in Woodland Hills, California

Julia Stone, in her 60s, raising four grandchildren in Los Angeles, California

Fay and Jim Strassburger, in their 60s, raising two grandsons in Los Angeles, California

Jane and Doug Sullivan, in their 60s, raising nine-year-old Elisa, five-year-old Shannon, and four-year-old Mark in Sherman Oaks, California

Alice Sutherland, in her 50s, raising 13-year-old Suzanne, 12-year-old Faith, and nine-year-old Tommy in Van Nuys, California

Anne Sutter, in her 60s, raising six-year-old Gregory in Long Beach, California

Arlene Townsend, in her 60s, raising seven-year-old Stuart in San Francisco, California

Rebecca Tybor, in her 70s, raising 16-year-old twins in Los Angeles, California

Grace and Marcus Tyler, in their 50s, raising five-year-old Jason in Pittsburgh, Pennsylvania

Dave and Milly Walsh, in their 70s, raising four grandchildren in Redondo Beach, California

John and Carol Waters, in their 60s, raising eight-year-old Brian in Long Beach, California

Notes

INTRODUCTION

1. Linda L. Creighton. "Silent Saviors," *U.S. News & World Report*, December 16, 1991, p. 83.
2. Mary Lou Wilson. "Recycled Parents," *The Reporter* (Vacaville, CA), March 19, 1990.
3. Andrew H. Malcolm. "Helping Grandparents Who Are Parents Again," *The New York Times*, November 19, 1991.
4. Lenora Madison Poe. *Black Grandparents as Parents.* Berkeley, CA: Lenora Madison Poe, 1992; Meredith Minkler and Kathleen M. Roe. *Grandmothers as Caregivers: Raising Children of the Crack Cocaine Epidemic.* Newbury Park, CA: Sage Publications, 1993; Irene M. Endicott. *Grandparenting Redefined: Guidance for Today's Changing Family.* Lynwood, WA: Aglow Publications, 1992.

CHAPTER 1

1. Jill Smolowe. "To Grandma's House We Go," *Time*, November 5, 1990, p. 90.
2. Ibid., p. 86; Meredith Minkler and Kathleen M. Roe. *Grandmothers as Caregivers: Raising Children of the Crack Cocaine Epidemic.* Newbury Park, CA: Sage Publications, 1993, pp. x, 4–5.
3. U.S. House of Representatives Select Committee on Aging. *Grandparents Rights: A Resource Manual.* Washington, DC: U.S. Government Printing Office, 1992, p. 15.
4. *Grandparent Information Center* (Handout). Washington, DC: AARP Grandparent Information Center.
5. *Grandparents Rights: A Resource Manual*, op. cit., p. 15.
6. Susan R. Pollack. "The Grandparent Trap," *The Detroit News*, July 17, 1991.

7. Mike Yorkey. "Picking Up the Pieces," *Focus on the Family*, September 1993, p. 13.

8. Patricia Edmonds. "Those Caught in Middle Are 'Missing a Lot,'" *USA Today*, July 23, 1991.

9. Laurie Becklund. "I Wanted Somebody to Love," *Los Angeles Times*, March 14, 1993; Center for the Study of Social Policy. *Kids Count Data Book: State Profiles of Child Well-Being*. Washington, DC: Annie E. Casey Foundation, 1993, p. 14.

10. Kristin A. Moore. *To Individuals and Organizations Concerned about Teen Pregnancy and Childbearing* (Memo). Washington, DC: Child Trends, February 1995.

11. U.S. Senate Committee on Labor and Human Resources. *Falling through the Crack: The Impact of Drug-Exposed Children on the Child Welfare System* (March 8, 1990). Washington, DC: U.S. Government Printing Office, 1990, p. 109.

12. Ellen Barry et al. *Manual for Grandparents and Caregivers* (3rd ed.). San Francisco: Legal Services for Prisoners with Children, 1993, p. 5.

13. *Falling through the Crack*, op. cit., pp. 18–21.

14. Ibid., p. 108.

15. Felicia R. Lee. "AIDS Toll on Elderly: Dying Grandchildren," *The New York Times*, November 21, 1994.

16. *Falling through the Crack*, op. cit., pp. 6, 9.

17. Interview with Mary Hayes (Division Chief, Foster Care Division, Department of Children and Family Services) by authors. Los Angeles, December 27, 1994.

18. There is no denying that the African American community is harder hit by the grandparenting phenomenon. According to the 1990 census, 12 percent of black children live with their grandparents, compared with four percent of white children. However, the actual *numbers* of black and white children are nearly equal: 1.2 million black children and 1.8 million white children. The discrepancy is due to the fact that there are five times more white children in the United States than black children. Hispanic children represent the smallest numbers, but they still number nearly half a million. See *Grandparents Rights: A Resource Manual*, p. 15.

19. Ibid., p. 15.

20. *Falling through the Crack*, op. cit., pp. 34, 161.

21. Ibid., p. 159.

22. Ibid., p. 94.

23. Karen Greene. "The Great American Grandparent: Reinventing Families," *Children's Advocate*, March/April 1992.

24. *Falling through the Crack*, op. cit., p. 36.

25. Interview with Michael Jones by authors (via telephone). June 22, 1994.

26. Linda L. Creighton. "Silent Saviors," *U.S. News & World Report*, December 16, 1991, p. 87.

CHAPTER 3

1. Andrew H. Malcolm. "Helping Grandparents Who Are Parents Again," *The New York Times*, November 19, 1991.
2. *Donahue*. April 11, 1991.
3. Susan R. Pollack. "The Grandparent Trap," *The Detroit News*, July 17, 1991.
4. Miriam Durkin. "When Grandparents Start Over," *Charlotte Observer*, November 3, 1991.
5. Tony Link. "When Kids Come to Grandma's House to Stay," *Daily News* (Los Angeles), December 19, 1989.
6. Laura Accinelli. "Starting Over," *Daily Breeze* (Torrance, California), September 11, 1988.
7. Madeleine Wild. "Grandmas Forced to Become Moms," *Woman's World*, July 16, 1991, p. 21.

CHAPTER 4

1. Eileen Beal. "Grandparents Raising Grandchildren," *Cleveland Jewish News*, November 23, 1990, p. 15.

CHAPTER 5

1. *Seniors Speak Out*, KPBS TV, San Diego, November 26, 1992.
2. Muriel Dobbin. "Grandmothers Fill In for Drug-Abusing Parents," *Senior Highlights*, March 1990, p. 5.
3. Harriet Goldhor Lerner. *The Dance of Intimacy*. New York: Harper & Row, 1989, p. 27.

CHAPTER 6

1. Robin Worthington. "The Second Time Around," *San Jose Mercury News*, March 22, 1992.
2. Sherry Angel. "Starting Over: Grandparents Who Step In and Raise Their Grandchildren," *Los Angeles Times/Orange County*, April 15, 1991.

3. Ingrid Watson. "Rocking the Cradle," *Fort Worth Star-Telegram*, November 13, 1988.
4. For a full definition of ADHD see: American Psychiatric Association. *Diagnostic and Statistical Manual of Mental Disorders* (4th ed.). Washington, DC: American Psyciatric Association, 1994, pp. 78–85.
5. Claudia Wallis. "Live in Overdrive," *Time*, July 28, 1994, p. 43.
6. Ibid., p. 43.
7. *Diagnostic and Statistical Manual of Mental Disorders*, op. cit.
8. Interview with Michael Jones by authors (via telephone). June 22, 1994.
9. Jane Glenn Haas. "It Can Be Grand to Be Raised by Grandparents," *The Orange County Register*, March 25, 1992.

CHAPTER 7

1. "General Information about Learning Disabilities." *National Information Center for Children and Youth with Disabilities. Fact Sheet Number 7* (FS7). Washington, DC: National Information Center for Children and Youth with Disabilities (NICHCY), 1993.
2. "Eight Famous Persons with Learning Disabilities," *Their World*, January 1981.

CHAPTER 8

1. Muriel Dobbins. "Grandmothers Fill In for Drug-Abusing Parents," *Senior Highlights*, March 1990, p. 5.
2. JoBeth McDaniel. "The Second Shift," *Life*, June 1, 1992, p. 65.
3. Thomas C. Holt, Eric Foner, and John A. Garraty, eds. *Reader's Companion to American History*. Boston: Houghton Mifflin Company, 1991, p. 297.
4. Ibid., p. 298.
5. Laura Feig. *Drug Exposed Infants and Children: Service Needs and Policy Questions*. Washington, DC: U.S. Department of Health and Human Services, 1990, p. 1; Interview with Jacqueline Battle, Infants of Substance Abusing Mothers Clinic, Los Angeles County–University of Southern California Medical Center, by authors. Los Angeles, October 1, 1993.
6. Information on the rise and effects of crack cocaine from : U.S. Senate Committee on Labor and Human Resources. *Children of Substance Abusers* (February 5, 1989). Washington, DC: U.S. Government Print-

ing Office, 1990; U.S. Senate Committee on Labor and Human Resources. *Falling through the Crack: The Impact of Drug-Exposed Children on the Child Welfare System* (March 8, 1990). Washington, DC: U.S. Government Printing Office, 1990; "Drugs and Narcotics," *Guide to American Law Supplement 1990.* St. Paul, MN: West Publishing Company, 1990, pp. 94–96.

7. *Falling through the Crack*, op. cit., pp. 18–19.
8. Anastasia Toufexis. "Innocent Victims," *Time*, May 13, 1991, p. 58.
9. *Falling through the Crack*, op. cit., p. 7.
10. Ibid., p. 65.
11. Ibid., p. 65.
12. Ibid., p. 96.
13. Ibid., p. 125.
14. Information on addiction has been adapted from several interviews and printed sources, including: *The Disease of Chemical Dependency.* Carson City, NV: Serenity Support Services, 1991; *What Everyone Should Know about Drug Abuse.* South Deerfield, MA: Channing L. Bete, 1990; *About Addiction.* South Deerfield, MA: Channing L. Bete, 1991.
15. "The Second Shift," op. cit., p. 66.
16. *Falling through the Crack*, op. cit., p. 58.
17. Ibid., p. 164.
18. *Donahue*, April 11, 1991.
19. "Drugs and Narcotics," op. cit., p. 95.
20. Interview with Jacqueline Battle, Infants of Substance Abusing Mothers, Los Angeles County–University of Southern California Medical Center, by authors. Los Angeles, October 1, 1993.
21. Interview with Dorsey Nunn, Legal Services for Prisoners with Children, by authors. Los Angeles, November 4, 1993.
22. *Falling through the Crack*, op. cit., p. 108.
23. *Children of Substance Abusers*, op. cit., p. 3.
24. *Falling through the Crack*, op. cit., p. 34.
25. Ibid., p. 95.
26. "Minimal Protocols for Response to Births Involving Indications of Prenatal Substance Abuse" (Memo from California Superior Court), January 31, 1994 (factsheet). Pasadena, CA: Open Arms Family Support Network, 1993; *Falling through the Crack*, op. cit., pp. 209–211; "Fetal Alcohol Syndrome," *Public Health Education Information Sheet.* White Plains, NY: March of Dimes Birth Defects Foundation, 1989.
27. Interview with Jacqueline Battle, op. cit.
28. Ibid.
29. Cathy Trost. "Born to Lose: Babies of Crack Users Crowd Hospitals, Break Everybody's Heart," *The Wall Street Journal*, July 18, 1989.
30. "Innocent Victims," op. cit., p. 59.

31. Interview with Fay Strassburger, California grandmother, by authors. Los Angeles, May 18, 1994.
32. Melissa Balmain Welner. "A Testament to Survival," *Orange County Register*, June 14, 1992.
33. Marie Kanne Poulsen. *Perinatal Substance Abuse: What's Best for the Children?* Garden Grove, CA: Orangewood Children's Foundation, 1992, p. 3.

CHAPTER 10

1. "Family 'Kin Care' Trend Increasing," *NASW News* (National Association of Social Workers), May 1992.
2. Trish Johnson. "'Older' Parents Need Support," *Katy Times*, February 25, 1990.
3. Interview with Ted Youmans, California attorney, by authors. Long Beach, California. October 22, 1993.
4. Ingrid Watson. "Rocking the Cradle," *Fort Worth Star-Telegram*, November 13, 1988.
5. Robin D. Leonard and Stephen Elias. *Family Law Dictionary*. Berkeley, CA: Nolo Press, 1990, p. 20.
6. Ibid., p. 44.
7. "Rocking the Cradle," op. cit.
8. Susan Swartz. "When Grandparents Are Parents Again," *Press-Democrat* (Santa Rosa, California). July 14, 1991.
9. Interview with Harold LaFlamme, California attorney, by authors. Buena Park, California, February 20, 1993.
10. Ibid.
11. Legal guardianship ends at age 18 in California; your state may differ.
12. Interview with Ted Youmans, California attorney, by authors. Santa Ana, California, March 6, 1993.
13. River Ginchild and Ellen Barry. *Manual for Grandparent–Relative Caregivers and Their Advocates*. San Francisco: Legal Services for Prisoners with Children, 1994, p. 10.
14. Ellen M. Barry et al. *Legal Manual for Children's Caregivers in Illinois*. San Francisco: Legal Services for Prisoners with Children and Chicago Legal Aid to Incarcerated Mothers, 1993, p. 1.
15. Ibid., p. 5.
16. See Lisa Goldoftaz and David Brown. *The Guardianship Book: How to Become a Child's Guardian in California* (revised). Berkeley, CA: Nolo Press, 1993.
17. Interview with Pamela Mohr, Executive Director, Alliance for Children's Rights, by authors. Los Angeles, May 10, 1994.

18. Judicial Council of California. *Guardianship Pamphlet*, p. 4.
19. Interview with Robert Walmsley, California attorney, by authors. Buena Park, California, February 20, 1993.
20. Ellen C. Segal and Naomi Karp. *Grandparent Visitation Disputes: A Legal Resource Manual*. Washington, DC: American Bar Association, 1989, p. 5. Additional information on grandparent visitation state by state is available in: U.S. House of Representatives Select Committee on Aging. *Grandparents Rights: A Resource Manual* (December 1992). Washington, DC: U.S. Government Printing Office, 1992, pp. 65–107. (This is a reprint of a 1991 report put out by the Congressional Resource Services, *CRS Report for Congress: Legal Overview of Grandparent Visitation Rights*, by Gina Marie Stevens and Gloria Sugars.
21. *Grandparents Rights: A Resource Manual*, op. cit., pp. 80–81.
22. Joan Schrager Cohen. *Helping Your Grandchildren through Their Parents' Divorce*. New York: Walker and Company, 1994, p. 132.
23. Interview with Michael Salazar, California attorney, by authors. Los Angeles, September 12, 1994.
24. Fran H. Zupan. "Love is Grand," *State Newspaper* (Columbia, South Carolina), April 9, 1992.
25. Interview with Michael Salazar, op. cit.
26. *Manual for Grandparent–Relative Caregivers and their Advocates*, op. cit., p. 24.
27. Interview with Charles Ollinger, Arizona attorney, by authors (via telephone). September 9, 1994.

CHAPTER 11

1. Interview with Ted Youmans, California attorney, by authors. Santa Ana, California, March 6, 1993.
2. Ibid.
3. Ibid.
4. Joan Schrager Cohen. *Helping Your Grandchildren through Their Parents' Divorce*. New York: Walker and Company, 1994, p. 139.
5. The petition of dependency must be filed within 48 hours in California. River Ginchild and Ellen Barry. *Manual for Grandparent–Relative Caregivers and Their Advocates*. San Francisco: Legal Services for Prisoners with Children, 1994, p. 29.
6. Social Security Act, Title IV-E, 42 USC 670 et seq., § 475. Note: The Federal Code uses the term *disposition hearing* for the establishment of a permanent plan; many states refer to this stage as the *permanent planning hearing*.

7. Interview with Pamela Mohr, Executive Director, Alliance for Children's Rights, by authors. Los Angeles, February 24, 1993.
8. 42 USC 670, op. cit.
9. Interview with Pamela Mohr, op. cit.
10. *Manual for Grandparent–Relative Caregivers and Their Advocates*, op. cit., p. 24.
11. Interview with Pamela Mohr, op. cit., March 29, 1994.
12. Interview with Charles Ollinger, Arizona attorney, by authors (via telephone). September 9, 1994.
13. Ibid.
14. Interview with Michael Salazar, California attorney, by authors. Los Angeles, September 12, 1994.
15. Interview with Pamela Mohr, op. cit.
16. Interview with Ted Youmans, op. cit.
17. Interview with Michael Salazar, California attorney, by authors. Buena Park, California, February 20, 1993.
18. Ellen Palmer. "Grandparents Raising Grandchildren—The Golden Years: Cancelled," *Valley Magazine* (Orange County Beach Cities, California). December 1990.
19. Ingrid Watson. "Rocking the Cradle," *Fort Worth Star-Telegram*, November 13, 1988.
20. Interview with Michael Salazar, op. cit., February 20, 1993.
21. U.S. Senate Committee on Labor and Human Resources. *Falling through the Crack: The Impact of Drug-Exposed Children on the Child Welfare System* (March 8, 1990). Washington, DC: U.S. Government Printing Office, 1990, p. 8.
22. Ibid., p. 58.
23. Interview with Ethel Dunn, Executive Director, Grandparents United for Children's Rights, by authors (via telephone). September 19, 1993.
24. Interview with Charles Ollinger, Arizona attorney, by authors. Long Beach, California. October 22, 1993.
25. Ibid.
26. Interview with John C. Wooley, California judge, by authors. Buena Park, California, February 20, 1993.
27. Interview with Charles Ollinger, Arizona attorney, by authors (via telephone). September 9, 1994.

CHAPTER 12

1. Miriam Durkin. "When Grandparents Start Over," *Charlotte Observer*, November 3, 1991.

2. Linda L. Creighton. "Silent Saviors," *U.S. News & World Report*, December 16, 1991, p. 80.
3. Michele L. Norris. "Grandmothers Who Fill Void Carved by Drugs," *Washington Post*, August 30, 1991.
4. These figures are based on 1989 maintenance benefits for children under the age of two in Missouri, multiplied by five. This is the minimum a family of five might have received in Missouri in 1989. U.S. House of Representatives Committee on Ways and Means. *Overview of Entitlement Programs: 1990 Green Book*. Washington, DC: U.S. Government Printing Office, 1990, p. 767.
5. *Overview of Entitlement Programs*, op. cit., pp. 556–557.
6. Interview with Pamela Mohr, Executive Director, Alliance for Children's Rights, by authors. Los Angeles, March 28, 1995.
7. River Ginchild and Ellen Barry. *Manual for Grandparent–Relative Caregivers and Their Advocates*. San Francisco: Legal Services for Prisoners with Children, 1994, p. 52.
8. Interview with Yolanda Vera, staff attorney for the National Health Law Program, by authors. Los Angeles, November 4, 1993.
9. *Aid to Families with Dependent Children (AFDC) Action Transmittal (No. ACF-AT-94-5)*. Washington, DC: U.S. Department of Health and Human Services, February 28, 1994.
10. Interview with Pamela Mohr, op. cit.
11. Foster care benefits are defined in Title IV-E of the Social Security Act, 42 USC 670 et seq., and are known as IV-E Foster Care. They may also be known as AFDC-FC (AFDC-Foster Care).
12. Legal Aid Foundation of Los Angeles Government Benefits Unit. *Foster Care Manual*. Los Angeles: Legal Aid Foundation of Los Angeles, 1993, p. 17; *Miller v. Youakim Fact Sheet*, photocopied.
13. *Foster Care Manual*, op. cit., pp. 15–16.
14. Jeffrey Miller. "Woman Fights Social Service Agencies," *Los Angeles Times*, January 3, 1988.
15. *Foster Care Manual*, op. cit., p. 29.
16. Social Security Administration. *Social Security and SSI Benefits for Children with Disabilities*. Baltimore: U.S. Department of Health and Human Services, Social Security Administration, 1993, p. 7.
17. Michele Melden. *An Introduction for Advocates to SSI for Children*. Los Angeles: The Alliance for Children's Rights, 1992, p. 13.
18. Ibid., p. 13.
19. *Social Security and SSI Benefits for Children with Disabilities*, op. cit., p. 9.
20. Interview with Pamela Mohr, op. cit.
21. Social Security Administration. *Survivors* (SSA Publication No. 05-10084). Baltimore: U.S. Department of Health and Human Services, Social Security Administration, 1993, p. 3.

22. Interview with Pamela Mohr, op. cit.
23. 42 U.S.C. § 1396d(r)(5) of the Medicaid Act. Cited in Jane Perkins. *Advocate's Medicaid EPSDT Reference Manual.* Chapel Hill, NC: National Health Law Program, 1993, p. 21.
24. Bonnie Armstrong. *An Agenda for Children's Health Care in Los Angeles County.* Los Angeles: Los Angeles Roundtable for Children, 1993.
25. Interview with Anne Rutherford, fiscal and program service coordinator, WIC, Portland, by authors (via telephone). August 30, 1993.

CHAPTER 13

1. Attributed to Walter Barbee. Source unknown.
2. "Legal Rights because of Learning Disabilities," *L/D Law,* 1990, p. 13.
3. Ibid., p. 13.
4. Rehabilitation Act of 1973. 29 USC 794 et seq., § 504, as explained in *L/D Law,* op. cit.
5. Individuals with Disabilities Education Act (Public Law 101-476) is an amendment of the Education for All Handicapped Act (Public Law 94-142). 20 USC 1401 et seq. in *NICHCY Briefing Paper: Individualized Education Programs (IEPs): Federal Regulations and Appendix C to Part 300.* Washington DC: National Information Center for Children and Youth with Disabilities (NICHCY), update March 1994.
6. Interview with Larry Hanna, California attorney, by authors. Los Angeles, May 13, 1993.
7. Pamela Darr Wright. *Your Child's IEP: Practical and Legal Guidance for Parents.* Richmond, VA: Pamela Darr Wright, Licensed Clinical Social Worker, 1994.
8. Interview with Peter Wright, Virginia attorney, by authors (via telephone). April 3, 1995.
9. Interview with Larry Hanna, California attorney, by authors. Sherman Oaks, California, August 11, 1993.
10. Interview with Peter Wright, Virginia attorney, by authors (via telephone). August, 1994.
11. Interview with Larry Hanna, op. cit., May 13, 1993.
12. *How to Participate in our Child's IEP Meeting.* Chicago, IL: Coordinating Council for Handicapped Children.
13. National Information Center for Children and Youth with Disabilities (NICHCY) *A Parent's Guide to Accessing Programs for Infants, Toddlers, and Preschoolers with Disabilities.* Washington, DC: NICHCY, 1992.
14. Interview with Larry Hanna, op. cit.

CHAPTER 14

1. Warren Harris. "Raising Second Family," *Las Vegas Sun*, June 19, 1989.
2. AARP Grandparent Information Center statistics, as of April 1994.
3. Catha McSweeney. "Filling the GAP," *Patriot Ledger*, October 27, 1989.

CHAPTER 15

1. "'Washington Summit' on Grandparent Caregiving," *Brookdale Grandparent Caregiver Information Project Newsletter*, February 1992, p. 2.
2. Senate Hearing: Joan McMillin (California) and Mary Ruth Shaheen (Maine) appeared before the U.S. Senate Special Committee on Aging on July 29, 1992. U.S. Senate Special Committee on Aging. *Grandparents as Parents: Raising a Second Generation* (July 29, 1992). Washington, DC: U.S. Government Printing Office, 1992, pp. 34, 37.
3. *Donahue*, April 11, 1991.
4. Sandy Pasqua. "Grandparents Mobilize to Demand Their Rights," *Senior World of Los Angeles*, September 1992.
5. Donna Kennedy. "When Grandparents Raise the Grandkids: 'Mrs. Rock' Battles to Change the Law," *Press-Enterprise* (Riverside, California), August 2, 1989.
6. In 1894 a Louisiana grandmother petitioned for visitation with her grandchildren, and lost, in the landmark case *Succession of Reiss*. The ruling supported the argument that grandparents' rights would interfere with parental rights and would undermine the parent's authority. Marie Purnell and Beatrice H. Bagby, "Grandparents Rights: Implications for Family Specialists," *Family Relations*, April 1993; Interview with Ethel Dunn, Executive Director, Grandparents United for Children's Rights, by authors (via telephone). September 19, 1993.
7. Interview with Ethel Dunn, op. cit.
8. U.S. House of Representatives Select Committee on Aging. *Grandparents Rights: A Resource Manual*. Washington, DC: U.S. Government Printing Office, 1992, pp. 1–2.
9. Interview with Ethel Dunn, op. cit., October 21, 1993.
10. Patty Housen. "Retiring to the Nursery: Grandparents Raising Kids' Kids," *Senior Beacon: In Focus for People Over 50*, May 1990, p. 1.
11. Interview with Michael Salazar, California attorney, by authors. Culver City, California, November 12, 1992.
12. U.S. House of Representatives Select Committee on Aging. *Grandparents Rights: Preserving Generational Bonds* (October 2, 1991). Washington, DC: U.S. Government Printing Office, 1991, p. 2.

13. Stephanie Edelstein. "Do Grandparents Have Rights?" *Modern Maturity*, December 1990–January 1991, p. 41–42.

14. Carolyn Pantier. "Many Grandparents Parenting Again," *Senior World of Los Angeles*, September 1993, p. 7.

15. Patrick Burke. "Grandfolks Win a Round," *Senior Spectrum*, August 1991, p. 1.

16. Patty Housen. "Retiring to the Nursery: Grandparents Raising Kids' Kids," *Senior Beacon: In Focus for People Over 50*, May 1990, p. 1; Interview with Barbara Kirkland, founder of Grandparents Raising Grandchildren, by authors (via telephone). April 11, 1994.

17. Act Regarding the Rights of Grandparents in Child Protection Proceedings, 22 MRSA 4005-B, § 1. (State of Maine)

18. Interview with Margie Davis, GOLD founder, by authors. Los Angeles, July 7, 1993.

19. Three hearings took place in the United States House and Senate between 1990 and 1992: "Grandparents Rights: Preserving Generational Bonds," House Select Committee on Aging, October 2, 1991; "Grandparents: New Roles and Responsibilities," House Select Committee on Aging, June 8, 1992; "Grandparents as Parents: Raising a Second Generation," Senate Special Committee on Aging, July 29, 1992.

20. "Coalitions Forming in Support of Grandparent Caregivers," *Brookdale Grandparent Caregiver Information Project Newsletter*, June 1992, p. 1.

21. "New Beginnings . . . The Grandparent Information Center Opens." *AARP Grandparent Information Center Newsletter*, Winter 1994, p. 1.

22. Interview with Ethel Dunn, op. cit.

23. Interview with Barbara Wasson, grandparent activist, by authors. Long Beach, California, March 2, 1994.

24. Interview with Rosalie Cauley, grandparent activist, by authors. Long Beach, California, October 21, 1993.

25. Margaret Collins. "Foster Parents a Safety Net," *Capital Times*, March 30, 1993.

26. Interview with Leza Davis, California legislative assistant, by authors (via telephone). October 30, 1994.

27. Interview with Margie Davis, op. cit., May 17, 1993.

28. Interview with Barbara Castro, grandparent activist, Long Beach, California, March 4, 1994.

29. *Grandparents Rights: A Resource Manual*, op. cit., p. 6.

30. Interview with Dr. Arthur Kornhaber, president and founder of the Foundation for Grandparenting, by authors (via telephone). March 23, 1995.

31. Interview with Margie Davis, op. cit., July 7, 1993.

CHAPTER 16

1. Alice Hornbaker. "Parents Second Time Around," *Cincinnati Enquirer*, September 10, 1991, p. 2.
2. Ethel Dunn. "Those Wonderful Abuelas," *Intergenerational Hookup*, Winter/Spring 1993, p. 1.
3. Reprinted with permission of Kevin de Toledo.
4. Donald O. Bolander, Dolores D. Varner, Gary B. Wright, and Stephanie H. Greene (compilers). *Instant Quotation Dictionary*. Little Falls, NJ: Career Publishing, 1981, p. 30.

Bibliography

BOOKS/MANUALS/HEARINGS

American Psychiatric Association. *Diagnostic and Statistical Manual of Mental Disorders* (4th ed.). Washington, DC: American Psychiatric Association, 1994.

Armstrong, Bonnie. *An Agenda for Children's Health Care in Los Angeles County.* Los Angeles: Los Angeles Roundtable for Children, 1993.

Barry, Ellen, David20 Fortier, Gail Smith, and Joanne Archibald. *Legal Manual for Children's Caregivers in Illinois.* San Francisco: Legal Services for Prisoners with Children and Chicago Legal Aid to Incarcerated Mothers, 1993.

Barry, Ellen, Dorsey Nunn, Carrie Kojimoto, Nancy Jacot-Bell, and Gabriela Lujan. *Manual for Grandparents and Caregivers* (3rd ed.). San Francisco: Legal Services for Prisoners with Children, 1993.

Center for the Study of Social Policy. *Kids Count Data Book: State Profiles of Child Well-Being.* Washington, DC: Annie E. Casey Foundation, 1993.

Cohen, Joan Schrager. *Helping Your Grandchildren through Their Parents' Divorce.* New York: Walker and Company, 1994.

Endicott, Irene M. *Grandparenting Redefined: Guidance for Today's Changing Family.* Lynwood, WA: Aglow Publications, 1992.

Ginchild, River, and Ellen Barry. *Manual for Grandparent–Relative Caregivers and Their Advocates.* San Francisco: Legal Services for Prisoners with Children, 1994.

The Guide to American Law Supplement 1990. St. Paul, MN: West Publishing Company, 1990.

Holt, Thomas C., Eric Foner, and John A. Garraty, eds. *Reader's Companion to American History.* Boston: Houghton Mifflin Company, 1991.

Keller, Helen. *We Bereaved.* New York: Leslie Fulenwider, 1929.

Leonard, Robin D., and Stephen Elias. *Family Law Dictionary.* Berkeley, CA: Nolo Press, 1990.

Lerner, Harriet Goldhor. *The Dance of Intimacy.* New York: Harper & Row, 1989.

Minkler, Meredith, and Kathleen M. Roe. *Grandmothers as Caregivers: Raising Children of the Crack Cocaine Epidemic.* Newbury Park, CA: Sage Publications, 1993.

Poe, Lenora Madison. *Black Grandparents as Parents.* Berkeley, CA: Lenora Madison Poe, 1992.

Segal, Ellen C., and Naomi Karp, eds. *Grandparent Visitation Disputes: A Legal Resource Manual.* Washington, DC: American Bar Association, 1989.

Tamborello, Frank, ed. *How to Get Food and Money in Los Angeles County.* Los Angeles, CA: Southern California Ecumenical Council Interface Hunger Coalition, 1993.

U.S. House of Representatives Committee on Ways and Means. *Overview of Entitlement Programs: 1990 Green Book.* Washington, DC: U.S. Government Printing Office, 1990.

U.S. House of Representatives Select Committee on Aging. *Grandparents: New Roles and Responsibilities* (June 8, 1992; Comm. Pub. No. 102-876). Washington, DC: U.S. Government Printing Office, 1992.

———. *Grandparents Rights: A Resource Manual* (December 1992; Comm. Pub. No. 102-898). Washington, DC: U.S. Government Printing Office, 1992.

———. *Grandparents Rights: Preserving Generational Bonds* (October 2, 1991; Comm. Pub. No. 102-833). Washington, DC: U.S. Government Printing Office, 1991.

U.S. Senate Committee on Labor and Human Resources. *Children of Substance Abusers* (February 5, 1989). Washington, DC: U.S. Government Printing Office, 1990.

———. *Falling Through the Crack: The Impact of Drug-Exposed Children on the Child Welfare System* (March 8, 1990). Washington, DC: U.S. Government Printing Office, 1990.

U.S. Senate Special Committee on Aging. *Grandparents as Parents: Raising a Second Generation* (July 29, 1992; Serial No. 102-24). Washington, DC: U.S. Government Printing Office, 1992.

BROCHURES/PAMPHLETS/PAPERS

About Addiction [Pamphlet].South Deerfield, MA: Channing L. Bete, 1991.

Advocacy . . . Why Bother? Sacramento, CA: On the Capitol Doorstep, 1989.

Aid to Families with Dependent Children (AFDC) Action Transmittal (No. ACF-AT-94-5). Washington, DC: U.S. Department of Health and Human Services, February 28, 1994.

Aid to Families with Dependent Children (AFDC) Fact Sheet. Sacramento, CA: Western Center on Law and Poverty, September 1991.

Alliance for Children's Rights. *A Manual on the Adoption Assistance Program.* Los Angeles: Alliance for Children's Rights, 1992. (Adapted from article by Alice Bussiere and Ellen C. Segal, "Adoption Assistance for Children with Special Needs" and a manual prepared by Pamela Mohr for the Children's Rights Project of Public Counsel).

———. *1992 Dependency Laws* (California). Los Angeles: Alliance for Children's Rights, October 1992. (Based on a manual by Pamela Mohr for the Children's Rights Project)

Anderson, Terry K., Susie Kaylor, and Joan Flaherty. *The Legislative Process: You Really Do Matter.* Sacramento, CA: Senate Select Committee on Citizen Participation in Government, 1989.

Barnes, Ellen. *IEP Checklist* (On-line). Syracuse, NY: Developmental Disabilities Rights Project and Direction Service Center on Human Policy, 1993. (Compuserve, ADD+ Forum, iepdoc.txt)

Battle, Jacqueline, Kathryn Payne, and Maureen S. Wilson. *Open Arms Baby Book: Special Care Techniques for Infants Prenatally Exposed to Drugs or Alcohol.* Pasadena, CA: Open Arms Family Support Network, 1995.

California Superior Court. *Minimal Protocols for Response to Births Involving Indications of Prenatal Substance Abuse* (Memo). January 31, 1994.

Coordinating Council for Handicapped Children. *How to Participate in our Child's IEP Meeting* (On-line). Chicago, IL: Coordinating Council for Handicapped Children, n.d. (Compuserve, ADD+ Forum, iep.txt)

Council for Exceptional Children and ERIC Clearinghouse on Handicapped and Gifted Children. *Providing an Appropriate Education to Children with Attention Deficit Disorder* (ERIC Digest No. E512) (On-line). Reston, VA: ERIC, Education Resources Information Center, 1992. (Compuserve, ADD+ Forum, appro.txt)

County of San Diego Department of Social Services. *Juvenile Dependency Court Information* (Brochure). San Diego: County of San Diego Department of Social Services, 1992.

———. *A Parent's Guide to Child Welfare Services* (Brochure). San Diego: County of San Diego Department of Social Services, October 1992.

Desk Guide: Rights and Responsibilities of Legal Guardians/Adoptive Parents (Handout). Los Angeles: County of Los Angeles Department of Children's Services, 1991.

Feig, Laura. *Drug Exposed Infants and Children: Service Needs and Policy Questions.* Washington, DC: U.S. Department of Health and Human Services, 1990.

"Fetal Alcohol Syndrome," *Public Health Education Information Sheet.* White Plains, NY: March of Dimes Birth Defects Foundation, 1989.

Finnegan, L. P., and B. A. Macnew, *American Journal of Nursing,* Vol 74., No. 4, April 1974. (As adapted in the handout "Comforting Techniques for an Infant Exposed to Drugs Prenatally," courtesy of Infants of Substance Abusing Mothers at Los Angeles County–University of Southern California Medical Center)

Fowler, Mary. *NICHCY Briefing Paper: Attention Deficit Disorder* (On-line). Washington, DC: National Information Center for Children and Youth with Disabilities (NICHCY), 1991. (Compuserve, ADD+ Forum, nbpadd.txt)

Frost, Diane, ed. *Children Who Learn Differently.* Sacramento, CA: California Association for Neurologically Handicapped Children (CANHC), Contra Costa West Chapter, 1975.

(Grandparent Information Center handout). Washington, DC: AARP Grandparent Information Center.

Grandparents Offering Love and Direction. *GOLD Court Assistance Program (CAP) for Relatives.* San Diego: Grandparents Offering Love and Direction, March 1992.

Grandparents Offering Love and Direction and San Diego County Department of Social Services. *Handbook for Relatives.* San Diego, CA: 1993.

Grandparents Rights: An Overview of the Law (Handout). Santa Ana, CA: Law Office of Van Deusen, Youmans and Walmsley, 1992.

Grandparents United for Children's Rights. *A Walk through Policyland: A How-To Manual on Dealing with Your Legislators.* Madison, WI: Grandparents United For Children's Rights, 1991.

Janov, Brooke. *AFDC, AFDC-FC, and Youakim Benefits: A Comparative Overview for Advocates and Clients.* Los Angeles: Alliance For Children's Rights, 1993.

Legal Aid Foundation of Los Angeles Government Benefits Unit. *The Foster Care Manual.* Los Angeles: Legal Aid Foundation of Los Angeles, 1993.

Lokerson, Jean. *Learning Disabilities* (ERIC Digest No. 516) (On-line). Reston, VA: Council for Exceptional Children, 1992. (Compuserve, ADD+ Forum, ericdi.ld)

Melden, Michele. *An Introduction for Advocates to SSI for Children.* Los Angeles: Alliance For Children's Rights, 1992.

Mental Health Law Project. *SSI: New Opportunities for Children with Disabilities, Checklists and Topic Sheets for Advocacy Training.* Washington, DC: Mental Health Law Project, 1991–1992.

Mohr, Pamela A., and Greg Bordo. *Legal Guardianship of the Person* (Draft). Los Angeles: Children's Rights Project, n.d.

Moore, Kristin A. *To Individuals and Organizations Concerned about Teen Pregnancy and Childbearing* (Memo). Washington, DC: Child Trends, February 1995.

Morgan, Daniel P. *Parents' Rights and Responsibilities* (On-line). Reston, VA: Educational Resource Information Center, 1984. (Compuserve, ADD+ Forum, right.txt)

National Information Center for Children and Youth with Disabilities. *Definition of Learning Disabilities* (Fact Sheet No. 7) (On-line). Washington, DC: National Information Center for Children and Youth with Disabilities (NICHCY), 1993. (Compuserve, ADD+ Forum, lddef.txt)

_____. *General Information about Public Agencies* (On-line). Washington, DC: National Information Center for Children and Youth with Disabilities (NICHCY), 1993. (Compuserve, ADD+ Forum, public.txt)

_____. *NICHCY Briefing Paper: Individualized Education Programs (IEPs): Federal Regulations and Appendix C to Part 300.* Washington, DC: National Information Center for Children and Youth with Disabilities (NICHCY), update March 1994.

_____. *NICHCY New Digest* (Vol. 1, No. 1). Washington, DC: National Information Center for Children and Youth with Disabilities (NICHCY), 1991.

_____. *NICHCY News Digest* (Vol. 3, No. 2). Washington, DC: National Information Center for Children and Youth with Disabilities (NICHCY), September 1993.

_____. *A Parent's Guide to Accessing Programs for Infants, Toddlers, and Preschoolers with Disabilities* (On-line). Washington, DC: National Information Center for Children and Youth with Disabilities (NICHCY), 1992. (Compuserve, ADD+ Forum, access.txt)

_____. *Questions Often Asked about Special Education Services* (Fact sheet). Washington, DC: National Information Center for Children and Youth with Disabilities (NICHCY), update 1993.

Perkins, Jane. *Advocate's Medicaid EPSDT Reference Manual.* Chapel Hill, NC: National Health Law Program, 1993.

Poulsen, Marie Kanne. *Perinatal Substance Abuse: What's Best for the Children?* Garden Grove, CA: Orangewood Children's Foundation, 1992.

Repetto, Jeanne, and Donna Wandry. *Transition Services in the IEP* (On-line). Washington, DC: National Information Center for Children and Youth with Disabilities (NICHCY), 1993. (Compuserve, ADD+ Forum, iep-1.txt)

Serenity Support Services. *The Disease of Chemical Dependency.* Carson City, NV: Serenity Support Services, 1991.

Social Security Administration. *Social Security and SSI Benefits for Children with Disabilities* (SSA Pub. No. 05-10026) (Brochure). Baltimore: U.S. Department of Health and Human Services, Social Security Administration, 1993.

_____. *SSI: Supplemental Security Income* (SSA Pub. No. 05-11000) (Brochure). Baltimore: U.S. Department of Health and Human Services, Social Security Administration, 1993.

_____. *Survivors* (SSA Pub. No. 05-10084) (Brochure). Baltimore: U.S. Department of Health and Human Services, Social Security Administration, 1993.

Stevens, Gina Marie, and Gloria Sugars. *CRS Report for Congress: Legal Overview of Grandparent Visitation Rights*. Washington, DC: Congressional Resource Services, 1991. (In U.S. House of Representatives Select Committee on Aging. *Grandparents Rights: A Resource Manual* [Comm. Pub. No. 102-898]. Washington, DC: U.S. Government Printing Office, 1992.

Vera, Yolanda. *Most Frequently Asked Questions Regarding Foster Care Children*. Los Angeles: Legal Aid Foundation of Los Angeles.

What Everyone Should Know about Drug Abuse (Pamphlet). South Deerfield, MA: Channing L. Bete Co., 1990.

Wright, Pamela Darr. *Your Child's IEP: Practical and Legal Guidance for Parents* (On-line). Richmond, VA: Pamela Darr Wright, 1994. (Compuserve, ADD+ Forum, ieps&c.txt)

MAGAZINES/NEWSPAPERS/JOURNALS

Accinelli, Laura. "Starting Over," *Daily Breeze* (Torrance, California), September 11, 1988.

Angel, Sherry. "Starting Over: Grandparents Who Step In and Raise Their Grandchildren, *Los Angeles Times/Orange County*, April 15, 1991.

Beal, Eileen. "Grandparents Raising Grandchildren," *Cleveland Jewish News*, November 23, 1990.

Becklund, Laurie. "I Wanted Somebody to Love," *Los Angeles Times*, March 14, 1993.

Burke, Patrick. "Grandfolks Win a Round," *Senior Spectrum*, August 1991.

"Coalitions Forming in Support of Grandpaent Caregivers," *Brookdale Grandparent Caregiver Information Project Newsletter*, June 1992.

Collins, Margaret. "Foster Parents a Safety Net," *Capital Times*, March 30, 1993.

Creighton, Linda L. "Silent Saviors," *U.S. News & World Report*, December 16, 1991.

Dobbin, Muriel. "Grandmothers Fill In for Drug-Abusing Parents," *Senior Highlights*, March 1990.

Dunn, Ethel. "Those Wonderful Abuelas," *Intergenerational Hookup*, Winter/Spring 1993.

Durkin, Miriam. "When Grandparents Start Over," *Charlotte Observer*, November 3, 1991.

Edelstein, Stephanie. "Do Grandparents Have Rights?" *Modern Maturity*, December 1990–January 1991.

Edmonds, Patricia. "Those Caught in Middle Are 'Missing a Lot,'" *USA Today*, July 23, 1991.

"Eight Famous Persons with Learning Disabilities," *Their World*, January 1981.

"Family 'Kin Care' Trend Increasing," *NASW News* (National Association of Social Workers), May 1992.

Greene, Karen. "The Great American Grandparent: Reinventing Families," *Children's Advocate*, March/April 1992.

Haas, Jane Glenn. "It Can Be Grand to Be Raised by Grandparents," *The Orange County Register*, March 25, 1992.

Harris, Warren. "Raising Second Family," *Las Vegas Sun*, June 19, 1989.

Hornbaker, Alice. "Parents Second Time Around," *Cincinnati Enquirer*, September 10, 1991.

Housen, Patty. "Retiring to the Nursery: Grandparents Raising Kids' Kids," *Senior Beacon: In Focus for People over 50*, May 1990.

Johnson, Trish. "'Older' Parents Need Support," *Katy Times*, February 25, 1990.

Kennedy, Donna. "When Grandparents Raise the Grandkids: 'Mrs. Rock' Battles to Change the Law," *Press-Enterprise* (Riverside, California), August 2, 1989.

Lee, Felicia R. "AIDS Toll on Elderly: Dying Grandchildren," *The New York Times*, November 21, 1994.

"Legal Rights because of Learning Disabilities," *L/D Law*, 1990.

Link, Tony. "When Kids Come to Grandma's House to Stay," *Daily News*, December 19, 1989.

Malcolm, Andrew H. "Helping Grandparents Who Are Parents Again," *The New York Times*, November 19, 1991.

McDaniel, JoBeth. "The Second Shift," *Life*, June 1, 1992.

McSweeny, Catha. "Filling the GAP," *Patriot Ledger*, October 27, 1989.

Miller, Jeffrey. "Woman Fights Social Service Agencies," *Los Angeles Times*, January 3, 1988.

"New Beginnings . . . The Grandparent Information Center Opens." *AARP Grandparent Information Center Newsletter*, Winter 1994.

Norris, Michele L. "Grandmothers Who Fill Void Carved by Drugs," *The Washington Post*, August 30, 1991.

Palmer, Ellen. "Grandparents Raising Grandchildren—The Golden Years: Cancelled," *Valley Magazine* (Orange County Beach Cities, California), December 1990.

Pantier, Carolyn. "Many Grandparents Parenting Again," *Senior World of Los Angeles*, September 1993.

Pasqua, Sandy. "Grandparents Mobilize to Demand Their Rights," *Senior World of Los Angeles*, September 1992.

Pollack, Susan R. "The Grandparent Trap," *The Detroit News*, July 17, 1991.

Purnell, Marie, and Beatrice H. Bagby, "Grandparents Rights: Implications for Family Specialists," *Family Relations*, April 1993.

Smolowe, Jill. "To Grandma's House We Go," *Time*, November 5, 1990.

Swartz, Susan. "When Grandparents Are Parents Again," *Press-Democrat*, (Santa Rosa, California), July 14, 1991.

Toufexis, Anastasia. "Innocent Victims," *Time*, May 13, 1991.

Trost, Cathy. "Born To Lose: Babies of Crack Users Crowd Hospitals, Break Everybody's Heart," *The Wall Street Journal*, July 18, 1989.

Wallis, Claudia. "Live in Overdrive," *Time*, July 28, 1994.

"'Washington Summit' on Grandparent Caregiving," *Brookdale Grandparent Caregiver Information Project Newsletter*, February 1992.

Watson, Ingrid. "Rocking the Cradle," *Fort Worth Star-Telegram*, November 13, 1988.

Welner, Melissa Balmain. "A Testament to Survival," *Orange County Register*, June 14, 1992.

Wilson, Mary Lou. "Recycled Parents," *The Reporter* (Vacaville, California), March 19, 1990.

Wild, Madeleine. "Grandmas Forced to Become Moms," *Woman's World*, July 16, 1991.

Worthington, Robin. "The Second Time Around," *San Jose Mercury News*, March 22, 1992.

Yorkey, Mike. "Picking Up the Pieces," *Focus on the Family*, September 1993.

Zupan, Fran H. "Love Is Grand," *State Newspaper* (Columbia, South Carolina), April 9, 1992.

MISCELLANEA

Social Security Act, Title IV-E, 42 USC 670 et seq., § 475.

Federal Register, Vol. 48, No. 100. May 23, 1983.

Rehabilitation Act of 1973. 29 USC 794 et seq., § 504.

Individuals with Disabilities Education Act (Public Law 101-476) (An amendment of Education for All Handicapped Act [Public Law 94-142]) 20 USC 1401 et seq.

Act Regarding the Rights of Grandparents in Child Protection Proceedings, 22 MRSA 4005-B, § 1. (State of Maine)

Donahue. April 11, 1991.

Seniors Speak Out, KPBS TV, San Diego, November 26 1992.

Index

AARP Grandparent Information Center (Washington, DC), 261, 279
Abandonment, 11, 13, 30, 67, 74, 79
  fear of, 73, 78
Acting out, 74, 77, 80, 103, 135
  sexually, 73, 100
  vs. verbalizing, 77, 81
Addiction, drug, 9, 11, 24, 30, 50, 61, 114–131
  and AIDS, 109
  as disease, 118–119
  history of, 115
  in middle class, 13
  and peer pressure, 128–129
  during pregnancy, 13
  preventing, 129–131
  and rehabilitation, 51–52, 117, 118
  treatment for, 51–52, 69
ADHD; *see* Attention-deficit/hyperactivity disorder
Adolescents, substance abuse in, 128–131
  warning signs of, 130
Adoption, 30, 67, 134, 145, 150, 154–156, 174
  assistance for, 155, 166, 210–213
  pressure for, 174–175
  and special needs children, 211
Adoption Assistance Program (AAP), 210–213
Adult children, 47–71; *see also* Siblings
  absence of, 10
  coping with, 50–51
  death of, 10, 11, 29, 30, 72, 75
  divorce of, 10, 11
  drug addiction in; *see* Addiction, drug
  dysfunctional, 29
  enabling, 51–52
  eviction of, 56–57

and financial support of children, 19, 69
  incarceration of, 11, 47, 63–65, 79
  manipulative, 49
  and repeat pregnancies, 49, 65–67
  return of children to, 132–138; *see also* Family reunification
  as single parents, 10
Advocacy, 18–19, 236
  political, 263–270, 273–274
AFDC; *see* Aid to Families with Dependent Children
African-American families, 13, 290*n*18
Aid to Families with Dependent Children (AFDC), 189, 192–198, 209; *see also* Foster care, Food stamps
  vs. foster care, 201
  and fraud, 198
  Immediate Need Cash program, 197
  linkage, 198, 199–200
  state involvement with, 192, 200
AIDS, 11, 93, 115, 273
Al-Anon, 54, 280
Alcohol abuse, 115, 116; *see also* Addiction
Alcoholics Anonymous, 64
Alliance for Children's Rights, 152
American Association of Retired Persons (AARP), 257, 261, 284
Anger, 28, 30–31
  of children, 61, 74, 76–77, 100
  effect of on marriage, 36
  expressing, 31, 77
Antidrug campaigns/groups, 131
Anxiety, 78
Appeal process
  in AFDC; *see* Aid to Families with Dependent Children
  in IEP; *see* Individual Education Program, appeal process; Special education

315